PSORIASIS DIET COOKBOOK

Complete Guide to Relief Including Anti inflammatory Recipes to Soothe your symptoms

TABLE OF CONTENTS

CHAPTER 1: INTRODUCTION

There lived a secret that afflicted the lives of many in the calm hamlet of Wellnessville where the murmurs of health-conscious citizens danced through the crisp air - an elusive ailment known as psoriasis. A culinary hero blossomed among the bustling farmers' markets and yoga studios. Enter the "Psoriasis Diet Cookbook," a gourmet excursion that promises more than just nutrition but also a path to breaking free from the chains of psoriasis. Join us on a delectable journey as we investigate the junction of nutrition and well-being, uncovering a symphony of ingredients that whisper the lovely song of healing. Welcome to the Wellnessville way of life, where each recipe is a step towards a better, more vibrant life.

ROLE OF DIET IN MANAGING PSORIASIS

Diet appears as a formidable companion in the management of psoriasis in the complicated tango between body and lifestyle. Join us on a trip where the plate is transformed into a canvas and each meal is a brushstroke that influences the skin's tale. As we delve into the science, we will uncover the impact of food choices on inflammation and skin regeneration. This investigation is about more than simply what's on your plate; it's about understanding the palette of nutrients that might contribute to a canvas of healthy skin. Welcome to the domain of food as medicine - an illuminating journey into the importance of diet in the delicate art of psoriasis management.

UNDERSTANDING PSORIASIS AND ITS TRIGGERS

Explore the intricate layers of the skin's tale, where psoriasis takes front stage. Unravel the intricacies of this perplexing state as we investigate its triggers, the elusive keys that allow it to exist. This investigation intends to shed light on the pathways that lead to psoriasis, from the intricate interplay of genetics to the dance of immunological responses. Join us as we unravel the complicated relationship between stress, lifestyle, and environmental variables, and see how these triggers are woven into the tapestry of skin health. Welcome to a comprehensive guide in which knowledge serves as a compass for navigating the complex terrain of understanding psoriasis and the numerous components that shape its story.

ANTI-INFLAMMATORY FOODS AND FOODS TO AVOID

Set out on a gastronomic trip that goes beyond taste, guiding you through a carefully curated selection of anti-inflammatory foods - the superheroes in your well-being quest. Discover the variety of nature's medicines from antioxidant-rich berries to the omega-3-rich embrace of fatty fish.

1. Fatty Fish (salmon, mackerel, sardines)
2. Berries (blueberries, strawberries, raspberries)
3. Leafy Greens (spinach, kale, Swiss chard)
4. Nuts and Seeds (almonds, walnuts, flaxseeds)
5. Olive Oil
6. Turmeric
7. Ginger
8. Green Tea
9. Avocado
10. Broccoli

Foods to Avoid for Inflammation:

1. Processed Sugars
2. Saturated Fats (found in red meat and full-fat dairy)
3. Trans Fats (found in some processed and fried foods)
4. Refined Carbohydrates (white bread, pastries, white rice)
5. Excessive Alcohol
6. Processed and Red Meat
7. High Sodium Foods (processed foods, canned soups)
8. Dairy (some individuals may be sensitive)
9. Artificial Additives and Preservatives
10. Nightshade Vegetables (some individuals may be sensitive, e.g, tomatoes, eggplants)

CHAPTER 2: BREAKFAST AND BEVERAGES

Quinoa Breakfast Bowl

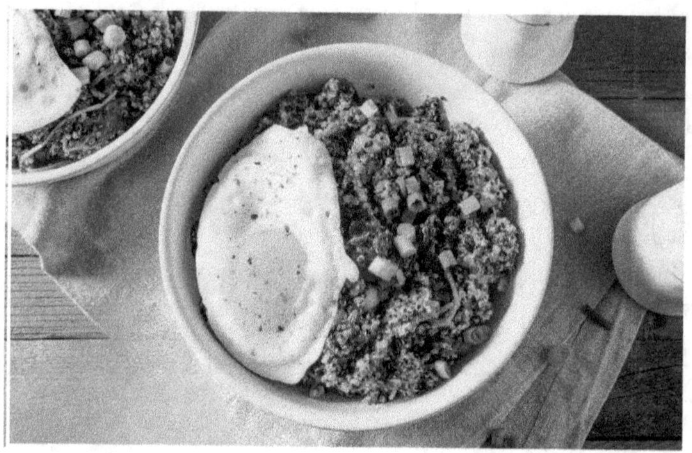

Ingredients:

- 1 cup quinoa, rinsed
- 2 cups water
- 1 tablespoon olive oil
- 1 small red onion, diced
- 2 cloves garlic, minced
- 1 cup cherry tomatoes, halved
- 1 cup spinach, chopped
- 1/2 cup cucumber, diced
- 1/4 cup fresh parsley, chopped
- 1/4 cup pumpkin seeds
- Salt and pepper to taste

Instructions:

1. In a medium saucepan, combine quinoa and water. Bring to a boil, then reduce heat, cover, and simmer for 15-20 minutes, or until quinoa is cooked and water is absorbed.

2. In a skillet, heat olive oil over medium heat. Add diced red onion and minced garlic, sautéing until softened.

3. Stir in cherry tomatoes and cook until they start to soften. Add chopped spinach and cook until wilted.

4. Fluff the cooked quinoa with a fork and add it to the skillet with the vegetables. Mix well to combine.

5. Add diced cucumber, fresh parsley, and pumpkin seeds to the skillet. Season with salt and pepper to taste. Continue to cook for a few more minutes until everything is heated through.

6. Serve the quinoa breakfast bowl warm, garnished with additional fresh parsley or a drizzle of olive oil if desired.

Avocado Toast with Smoked Salmon:

Ingredients:

- 2 slices whole-grain bread
- 1 ripe avocado
- 1 tablespoon lemon juice
- Salt and pepper to taste
- 4 ounces smoked salmon
- 1 tablespoon capers
- Fresh dill for garnish (optional)

Instructions:

1. Toast the whole-grain bread slices to your liking.

2. While the bread is toasting, mash the ripe avocado in a bowl. Add lemon juice, salt, and pepper to taste. Mix well.

3. Once the bread is toasted, spread the mashed avocado evenly over each slice.

4. Place smoked salmon on top of the avocado-covered toast.

5. Sprinkle capers over the smoked salmon for added flavor.

6. Optionally, garnish with fresh dill for a burst of herbal freshness.

7. Serve the avocado toast with smoked salmon immediately for a delicious and nutritious meal.

Chia Seed Pudding:

Ingredients:

- 1/4 cup chia seeds
- 1 cup almond milk (or any milk of your choice)
- 1 tablespoon maple syrup or honey
- 1/2 teaspoon vanilla extract
- Fresh fruits or berries for topping (optional)
- Nuts or granola for added crunch (optional)

Instructions:

1. In a bowl, combine chia seeds, almond milk, maple syrup or honey, and vanilla extract.

2. Whisk the mixture thoroughly to ensure the chia seeds are evenly distributed and don't clump together.

3. Cover the bowl and refrigerate for at least 2 hours or overnight. Stir the mixture after the first 15 minutes to prevent clumping.

4. Once the chia pudding has thickened to your desired consistency, give it a final stir.

5. Serve the chia seed pudding in individual bowls or jars.

6. Top with fresh fruits, berries, nuts, or granola for added texture and flavor.

7. Enjoy the chia seed pudding as a healthy and satisfying breakfast or snack.

Sweet Potato and Spinach Frittata:

Ingredients:

- 1 large sweet potato, peeled and thinly sliced
- 1 cup fresh spinach, chopped
- 8 large eggs
- 1/2 cup milk
- 1/2 cup shredded cheddar cheese
- 1 small onion, finely chopped
- 2 cloves garlic, minced
- 2 tablespoons olive oil
- Salt and pepper to taste
- Fresh herbs for garnish (e.g., parsley or chives)

Instructions:

1. Preheat the oven to 375°F (190°C).
2. In a large oven-safe skillet, heat olive oil over medium heat. Add chopped onions and minced garlic, sautéing until softened.
3. Add sweet potato slices to the skillet and cook until they start to become tender, about 5-7 minutes.
4. Stir in chopped spinach and cook until wilted.
5. In a bowl, whisk together eggs, milk, salt, and pepper.
6. Pour the egg mixture over the vegetables in the skillet. Allow it to set for a minute without stirring.
7. Sprinkle shredded cheddar cheese evenly over the egg mixture.
8. Transfer the skillet to the preheated oven and bake for 15-20 minutes or until the frittata is set in the center.
9. Once cooked, remove the skillet from the oven and let the frittata cool for a few minutes.
10. Garnish with fresh herbs and slice into wedges.
11. Serve the sweet potato and spinach frittata warm, either as a main dish or a hearty brunch option.

Oatmeal with Berries and Almonds:

Ingredients:

- 1 cup old-fashioned oats
- 2 cups milk (dairy or plant-based)
- 1 cup mixed berries (strawberries, blueberries, raspberries)
- 2 tablespoons sliced almonds
- 1 tablespoon honey or maple syrup
- 1/2 teaspoon vanilla extract
- Pinch of salt

Instructions:

1. In a saucepan, bring the milk to a simmer over medium heat.
2. Stir in the old-fashioned oats and reduce the heat to low. Cook, stirring occasionally, for about 5-7 minutes or until the oats are creamy and have absorbed the liquid.
3. Add a pinch of salt, vanilla extract, and honey or maple syrup to the oatmeal. Stir well to combine.
4. Remove the saucepan from the heat and let it sit for a minute to thicken.
5. In serving bowls, top the oatmeal with mixed berries and sliced almonds.
6. Drizzle a little extra honey or maple syrup over the berries and almonds for sweetness.
7. Serve the oatmeal with berries and almonds warm, and enjoy a wholesome and nutritious breakfast.

Greek Yogurt Parfait:

Ingredients:

- 1 cup Greek yogurt
- 1 cup granola
- 1 cup mixed berries (strawberries, blueberries, raspberries)
- 2 tablespoons honey

- 1/4 cup chopped nuts (e.g., almonds, walnuts)
- Fresh mint leaves for garnish (optional)

Instructions:

1. In a glass or bowl, start by layering about 1/4 cup of Greek yogurt at the bottom.
2. Add a layer of granola on top of the yogurt.
3. Place a layer of mixed berries over the granola.
4. Drizzle honey over the berries to add sweetness.
5. Repeat the layers until you fill the glass or bowl, finishing with a dollop of Greek yogurt on top.
6. Sprinkle chopped nuts over the final layer for added crunch and protein.
7. Garnish with fresh mint leaves if desired.
8. Serve the Greek yogurt parfait immediately as a delicious and nutritious breakfast, snack, or dessert.

Egg and Veggie Muffins:

Ingredients:

- 6 large eggs
- 1/2 cup diced bell peppers (any color)
- 1/2 cup diced tomatoes
- 1/2 cup diced spinach
- 1/4 cup diced red onion
- 1/4 cup shredded cheese (cheddar or your choice)
- Salt and pepper to taste
- Cooking spray or olive oil for greasing

Instructions:

1. Preheat the oven to 350°F (175°C).
2. In a bowl, whisk the eggs until well beaten. Season with salt and pepper.
3. Grease a muffin tin with cooking spray or a small amount of olive oil.

4. Divide the diced bell peppers, tomatoes, spinach, and red onion evenly among the muffin tin cups.

5. Pour the beaten eggs over the vegetables in each cup, filling about 3/4 full.

6. Sprinkle shredded cheese on top of each egg and veggie mixture.

7. Bake in the preheated oven for 18-20 minutes or until the egg muffins are set and slightly golden on top.

8. Allow the muffins to cool for a few minutes before gently removing them from the muffin tin.

9. Serve the egg and veggie muffins warm, either as a grab-and-go breakfast or a protein-packed snack.

Coconut Flour Pancakes:

Ingredients:

- 1/2 cup coconut flour
- 1/2 teaspoon baking powder
- Pinch of salt
- 4 large eggs
- 1 cup coconut milk (or any milk of your choice)
- 2 tablespoons melted coconut oil (plus extra for cooking)
- 1 tablespoon honey or maple syrup
- 1 teaspoon vanilla extract

Instructions:

1. In a bowl, whisk together the coconut flour, baking powder, and a pinch of salt.

2. In a separate bowl, beat the eggs. Add coconut milk, melted coconut oil, honey or maple syrup, and vanilla extract. Mix well.

3. Pour the wet ingredients into the bowl with the dry ingredients. Stir until just combined. Let the batter sit for a few minutes to allow the coconut flour to absorb the liquids.

4. Heat a skillet or griddle over medium heat. Grease with coconut oil.

5. Spoon about 1/4 cup of batter onto the hot skillet for each pancake.

6. Cook until bubbles form on the surface, then flip and cook the other side until golden brown.

7. Repeat until all the batter is used, adding more coconut oil to the skillet as needed.

8. Serve the coconut flour pancakes warm, topped with your favorite fruits, nuts, or a drizzle of honey.

Spinach and Mushroom Omelette:

Ingredients:

- 3 large eggs
- 1 cup fresh spinach, chopped
- 1/2 cup mushrooms, sliced
- 1/4 cup shredded cheese (e.g., feta, cheddar)
- 1/4 cup diced onion
- 1 clove garlic, minced
- 1 tablespoon olive oil
- Salt and pepper to taste
- Fresh herbs for garnish (e.g., parsley or chives)

Instructions:

1. In a bowl, whisk the eggs until well beaten. Season with salt and pepper.

2. Heat olive oil in a non-stick skillet over medium heat.

3. Add diced onions and minced garlic to the skillet, sautéing until softened.

4. Add sliced mushrooms to the skillet and cook until they release their moisture and become tender.

5. Stir in the chopped spinach and cook until wilted.

6. Pour the beaten eggs over the vegetable mixture in the skillet.

7. Allow the eggs to set for a moment, then gently lift the edges with a spatula, tilting the skillet to let any uncooked egg flow underneath.

8. Sprinkle shredded cheese over one half of the omelette.

9. Once the eggs are mostly set but still slightly runny on top, carefully fold the omelette in half using the spatula.

10. Continue cooking for another minute or until the cheese is melted and the omelette is cooked through.

11. Slide the omelette onto a plate and garnish with fresh herbs.

12. Serve the spinach and mushroom omelette hot, and enjoy a nutritious and flavorful meal.

Banana Walnut Smoothie:

Ingredients:

- 1 ripe banana
- 1/2 cup Greek yogurt
- 1/2 cup milk (dairy or plant-based)
- 1/4 cup chopped walnuts
- 1 tablespoon honey or maple syrup (optional, depending on sweetness preference)
- 1/2 teaspoon vanilla extract
- Ice cubes (optional)

Instructions:

1. Peel the ripe banana and place it in a blender.

2. Add Greek yogurt, milk, chopped walnuts, honey or maple syrup (if using), and vanilla extract to the blender.

3. If you prefer a colder smoothie, you can add a handful of ice cubes.

4. Blend all the ingredients until smooth and creamy.

5. Taste the smoothie and adjust sweetness or thickness by adding more honey, maple syrup, or milk if needed.

6. Pour the banana walnut smoothie into a glass.

7. Optionally, garnish with a sprinkle of chopped walnuts on top.

8. Serve the smoothie immediately for a delicious and nutrient-packed drink.

Buckwheat Pancakes with Blueberry Compote:

Ingredients:

- 1 cup buckwheat flour
- 1 tablespoon sugar
- 1 teaspoon baking powder
- 1/2 teaspoon baking soda
- 1/4 teaspoon salt
- 1 cup buttermilk
- 1 large egg
- 2 tablespoons melted butter (plus extra for cooking)
- 1 teaspoon vanilla extract

Instructions:

1. In a large bowl, whisk together buckwheat flour, sugar, baking powder, baking soda, and salt.
2. In a separate bowl, whisk together buttermilk, egg, melted butter, and vanilla extract.
3. Pour the wet ingredients into the bowl with the dry ingredients. Stir until just combined. Let the batter rest for a few minutes.
4. Heat a skillet or griddle over medium heat. Grease with butter.
5. Spoon about 1/4 cup of batter onto the hot skillet for each pancake.
6. Cook until bubbles form on the surface, then flip and cook the other side until golden brown.
7. Repeat until all the batter is used, adding more butter to the skillet as needed.

Blueberry Compote:

Ingredients:

- 1 cup blueberries
- 2 tablespoons sugar
- 1 tablespoon water
- 1/2 teaspoon lemon zest

- 1 tablespoon lemon juice

Instructions:

1. In a saucepan, combine blueberries, sugar, water, lemon zest, and lemon juice.
2. Bring the mixture to a simmer over medium heat, stirring occasionally.
3. Simmer for 8-10 minutes or until the blueberries break down and the compote thickens slightly.
4. Remove from heat and let it cool slightly.

Beverages:

Green Tea Lemonade:

Ingredients:

- 2 green tea bags
- 2 cups hot water
- 1/4 cup honey or agave syrup (adjust to taste)
- 1/2 cup freshly squeezed lemon juice (about 3-4 lemons)
- Ice cubes
- Lemon slices and mint leaves for garnish (optional)

Instructions:

1. Brew Green Tea:
   - Place green tea bags in a heatproof container.
   - Pour hot water over the tea bags.
   - Steep for 3-5 minutes, depending on your desired strength.
   - Remove the tea bags and allow the tea to cool to room temperature.
2. Sweeten the Tea:
   - Stir in honey or agave syrup into the cooled green tea until well dissolved.
3. Add Lemon Juice:
   - Squeeze fresh lemons to obtain 1/2 cup of lemon juice.
   - Add the lemon juice to the sweetened green tea and stir well.

4. Chill the Mixture:

   o Place the green tea lemonade in the refrigerator to chill for at least 1-2
     hours.

5. Serve:

   o Fill glasses with ice cubes.

   o Pour the chilled green tea lemonade over the ice.

Turmeric Golden Milk:

Ingredients:
- 2 cups milk (dairy or plant-based)
- 1 teaspoon ground turmeric
- 1/2 teaspoon ground cinnamon
- 1/4 teaspoon ground ginger
- 1/4 teaspoon ground cardamom
- 1 pinch black pepper (enhances turmeric absorption)
- 1 tablespoon honey or maple syrup (adjust to taste)
- 1 teaspoon coconut oil (optional)
- 1/2 teaspoon vanilla extract (optional)

Instructions:
1. Combine Ingredients:
   o In a saucepan, combine milk, ground turmeric, ground cinnamon, ground
     ginger, ground cardamom, and a pinch of black pepper.
2. Heat the Mixture:
   o Heat the mixture over medium heat, stirring constantly to avoid sticking.
3. Add Sweetener:
   o Once the milk is warm, add honey or maple syrup. Adjust sweetness to
     your liking.
4. Optional Additions:
   o Stir in coconut oil and vanilla extract if desired. These add depth and
     richness to the golden milk.
5. Simmer:
   o Allow the mixture to simmer for about 5 minutes, ensuring it doesn't come
     to a boil.
6. Strain (Optional):

- If you prefer a smoother consistency, you can strain the golden milk using a fine mesh sieve or cheesecloth.
7. Serve:
    - Pour the turmeric golden milk into mugs.

Cucumber Mint Infused Water:

Ingredients:
- 1 medium cucumber, thinly sliced
- Handful of fresh mint leaves
- 1-2 liters of water (depending on desired strength)
- Ice cubes (optional)

Instructions:
1. Prepare Ingredients:
    - Wash the cucumber thoroughly and slice it thinly.
    - Wash the mint leaves.
2. Combine Ingredients:
    - In a large pitcher, combine the cucumber slices and fresh mint leaves.
3. Muddle (Optional):
    - If you want a more intense flavor, gently muddle the cucumber and mint with a muddler or the back of a spoon. This helps release their natural flavors.
4. Add Water:
    - Pour the water over the cucumber and mint in the pitcher.
5. Refrigerate:
    - Place the pitcher in the refrigerator and let it chill for at least 2 hours to allow the flavors to infuse.
6. Serve:
    - Pour the cucumber mint infused water into glasses over ice cubes if desired.

Berry Blast Smoothie:

Ingredients:
- 1 cup mixed berries (strawberries, blueberries, raspberries)
- 1/2 banana, frozen
- 1/2 cup Greek yogurt
- 1/2 cup almond milk (or any milk of your choice)
- 1 tablespoon honey or maple syrup (optional, depending on sweetness preference)

- 1/2 teaspoon chia seeds (optional)
- Ice cubes (optional)

Instructions:

1. Prepare Ingredients:
   - If using fresh berries, wash them thoroughly. If the banana is not frozen, you can add ice cubes later for a colder smoothie.
2. Combine in Blender:
   - Place the mixed berries, frozen banana, Greek yogurt, almond milk, and honey or maple syrup in a blender.
3. Optional Additions:
   - If you want to boost the nutritional content, add chia seeds to the blender.
4. Blend Until Smooth:
   - Blend all the ingredients until smooth and creamy. If the consistency is too thick, you can add more almond milk.
5. Taste and Adjust:
   - Taste the smoothie and adjust sweetness or thickness by adding more honey, maple syrup, or milk if needed.
6. Serve:
   - Pour the Berry Blast Smoothie into a glass.

Pineapple Ginger Wellness Juice:

Ingredients:

- 2 cups fresh pineapple chunks
- 1-inch piece of ginger, peeled and sliced
- 1 lemon, juiced
- 1 tablespoon honey (optional)
- 2 cups cold water
- Ice cubes (optional)

Instructions:

1. Place the fresh pineapple chunks and ginger slices in a blender.
2. Squeeze the juice from the lemon into the blender.
3. Add honey if desired for sweetness.
4. Pour in cold water to the blender.

5. Blend the ingredients until smooth.

6. Strain the juice using a fine mesh sieve or cheesecloth to remove pulp.

7. Pour the strained juice into a glass over ice cubes if desired.

8. Garnish with a pineapple wedge or a slice of ginger.

9. Stir well before serving.

Herbal Chamomile Tea:

Ingredients:

- 1 chamomile tea bag or 1 tablespoon dried chamomile flowers
- 1 cup boiling water
- 1 teaspoon honey (optional)
- Lemon wedge (optional)

Instructions:

1. Place the chamomile tea bag or dried chamomile flowers in a teapot or mug.

2. Pour boiling water over the chamomile.

3. Let it steep for 5-7 minutes to allow the flavors to infuse.

4. Remove the tea bag or strain out the chamomile flowers.

5. Add honey if you prefer a sweeter taste.

6. Stir well and adjust sweetness to your liking.

7. Squeeze a lemon wedge into the tea for a citrusy twist if desired.

8. Serve and enjoy the soothing and calming effects of herbal chamomile tea.

Beetroot and Carrot Juice:

Ingredients:

- 2 medium-sized beetroots, peeled and chopped
- 3 medium-sized carrots, peeled and sliced
- 1 apple, cored and chopped
- 1-inch piece of ginger, peeled
- 1 lemon, juiced

- 2 cups cold water
- Ice cubes (optional)

Instructions:

1. Place the chopped beetroots, sliced carrots, chopped apple, and peeled ginger in a blender.
2. Squeeze the juice from the lemon into the blender.
3. Add cold water to the blender.
4. Blend the ingredients until smooth.
5. Strain the juice using a fine mesh sieve or cheesecloth to remove pulp.
6. Pour the strained juice into a glass over ice cubes if desired.
7. Stir well before serving.

Sparkling Lemon Basil Water:

Ingredients:

- 1 lemon, thinly sliced
- Fresh basil leaves (about 10-12 leaves)
- 2 cups sparkling water
- Ice cubes
- Optional: Sweetener of your choice (such as honey or agave syrup)

Instructions:

1. Place the lemon slices and fresh basil leaves in a pitcher.
2. Pour sparkling water over the lemon and basil.
3. Add ice cubes to the pitcher for a refreshing chill.
4. If desired, add a sweetener of your choice to taste and stir well.
5. Allow the flavors to infuse for about 10-15 minutes.
6. Pour the sparkling lemon basil water into glasses.
7. Garnish with additional lemon slices or basil leaves if desired.

Aloe Vera Citrus Cooler:

Ingredients:

- 1 cup fresh aloe vera gel (scooped from aloe leaves)
- 1 orange, juiced
- 1 lime, juiced
- 1 tablespoon honey or agave syrup (optional)
- 2 cups cold water
- Ice cubes

Instructions:

1. Scoop out 1 cup of fresh aloe vera gel from aloe leaves.
2. In a blender, combine the aloe vera gel, orange juice, lime juice, and honey (if using).
3. Add cold water to the blender.
4. Blend the ingredients until well combined and smooth.
5. Strain the mixture using a fine mesh sieve to remove any pulp.
6. Pour the strained Aloe Vera Citrus Cooler into a pitcher.
7. Chill in the refrigerator for at least 30 minutes.
8. Serve over ice cubes in glasses.

Matcha Latte:

Ingredients:

- 1 teaspoon matcha powder
- 1 tablespoon hot water
- 1 cup milk (dairy or plant-based)
- 1-2 teaspoons sweetener of choice (such as honey or agave syrup)
- Optional: Vanilla extract for added flavor

Instructions:

1. In a bowl, whisk together the matcha powder and hot water until a smooth paste forms.

2. Heat the milk in a saucepan or microwave until hot but not boiling.

3. Pour the hot milk over the matcha paste.

4. Add sweetener to taste and optional vanilla extract.

5. Use a frother or whisk to froth the matcha latte until it becomes creamy and foamy.

6. Pour the matcha latte into a cup.

7. Optional: Dust the top with a sprinkle of matcha powder.

8. Enjoy your comforting and energizing Matcha Latte!

Pomegranate Iced Tea:

Ingredients:

- 2 black tea bags
- 2 cups boiling water
- 1/2 cup pomegranate juice
- 2 tablespoons honey or sweetener of choice (adjust to taste)
- Ice cubes
- Fresh mint leaves for garnish (optional)
- Pomegranate arils for garnish (optional)

Instructions:

1. Place the black tea bags in a heatproof pitcher.

2. Pour boiling water over the tea bags and steep for 3-5 minutes.

3. Remove the tea bags and allow the tea to cool to room temperature.

4. Stir in the pomegranate juice and honey until well combined.

5. Refrigerate the tea for at least 1 hour to chill.

6. Fill glasses with ice cubes.

7. Pour the chilled Pomegranate Iced Tea into the glasses.

8. Garnish with fresh mint leaves and pomegranate arils if desired.

9. Stir before sipping to blend the flavors.

Quinoa Salad with Grilled Vegetables:

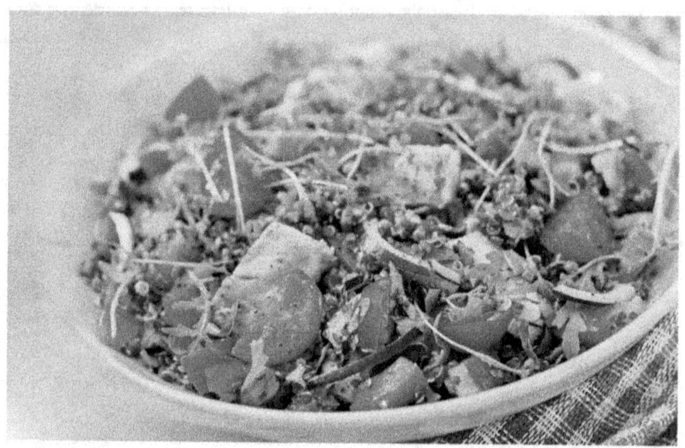

Ingredients:

- 1 cup quinoa, rinsed
- 2 cups water or vegetable broth
- 1 red bell pepper, sliced
- 1 zucchini, sliced
- 1 yellow squash, sliced
- 1 red onion, thinly sliced
- 1 cup cherry tomatoes, halved
- 3 tablespoons olive oil
- 2 tablespoons balsamic vinegar
- 1 teaspoon Dijon mustard
- Salt and pepper to taste
- Fresh herbs (such as parsley or basil) for garnish

Instructions:

1. In a saucepan, combine quinoa and water or vegetable broth. Bring to a boil, then reduce heat, cover, and simmer for 15-20 minutes until quinoa is cooked and water is absorbed. Fluff with a fork and let it cool.
2. Preheat the grill or grill pan over medium-high heat.
3. In a bowl, toss the sliced bell pepper, zucchini, yellow squash, and red onion with 2 tablespoons of olive oil. Season with salt and pepper.
4. Grill the vegetables for 4-5 minutes on each side or until they have nice grill marks and are tender.
5. In a small bowl, whisk together the remaining 1 tablespoon of olive oil, balsamic vinegar, Dijon mustard, salt, and pepper to create the dressing.
6. In a large bowl, combine the cooked quinoa, grilled vegetables, cherry tomatoes, and the dressing. Toss gently to combine.
7. Garnish with fresh herbs before serving.

Salmon and Avocado Wrap:

Ingredients:

- 2 salmon fillets, grilled or baked
- 2 whole-grain wraps or tortillas
- 1 avocado, sliced
- 1 cup mixed salad greens (e.g., spinach, arugula)
- 1/4 cup cherry tomatoes, halved
- 2 tablespoons Greek yogurt or sour cream
- 1 tablespoon lemon juice
- Salt and pepper to taste
- Optional: Red onion slices, cucumber strips, or your favorite salsa for additional toppings

Instructions:

1. Grill or bake the salmon fillets until cooked through.

2. In a small bowl, mix Greek yogurt or sour cream with lemon juice. Season with salt and pepper to taste.

3. Lay out the whole-grain wraps on a clean surface.

4. Spread a portion of the yogurt or sour cream mixture onto each wrap.

5. Place a grilled salmon fillet in the center of each wrap.

6. Top the salmon with sliced avocado, mixed salad greens, and cherry tomatoes.

7. If desired, add additional toppings like red onion slices, cucumber strips, or salsa.

8. Fold the sides of the wrap and roll it up tightly.

9. Secure the wraps with toothpicks if needed.

10. Slice the wraps in half diagonally before serving.

Mediterranean Chickpea Bowl:

Ingredients:

- 1 cup cooked quinoa or couscous
- 1 can (15 oz) chickpeas, drained and rinsed
- 1 cup cherry tomatoes, halved
- 1 cucumber, diced
- 1/2 red onion, finely chopped
- 1/2 cup Kalamata olives, sliced
- 1/2 cup crumbled feta cheese
- 2 tablespoons olive oil
- 1 tablespoon balsamic vinegar
- 1 teaspoon dried oregano
- Salt and pepper to taste
- Fresh parsley for garnish

Instructions:

1. In a large bowl, combine cooked quinoa or couscous, chickpeas, cherry tomatoes, cucumber, red onion, Kalamata olives, and feta cheese.

2. In a small bowl, whisk together olive oil, balsamic vinegar, dried oregano, salt, and pepper to create the dressing.

3. Pour the dressing over the chickpea mixture and toss gently to combine.

4. Garnish with fresh parsley.

5. Serve the Mediterranean Chickpea Bowl immediately or refrigerate for a chilled option.

Turkey and Hummus Wrap:

Ingredients:

- 2 whole-grain wraps or tortillas
- 1/2 pound (about 225g) thinly sliced turkey breast
- 1/2 cup hummus
- 1 cup mixed salad greens (e.g., spinach, arugula)
- 1 cucumber, thinly sliced
- 1 tomato, sliced
- 1/4 red onion, thinly sliced
- 1 tablespoon olive oil
- 1 tablespoon lemon juice
- Salt and pepper to taste

Instructions:

1. Lay out the whole-grain wraps on a clean surface.

2. Spread a generous layer of hummus onto each wrap.

3. Place a portion of thinly sliced turkey breast on top of the hummus.

4. In a bowl, toss the mixed salad greens, cucumber slices, tomato slices, and red onion with olive oil and lemon juice. Season with salt and pepper to taste.

5. Distribute the salad mixture evenly over the turkey on each wrap.

6. Fold the sides of the wraps and roll them up tightly.

7. Secure the wraps with toothpicks if needed.

8. Slice the wraps in half diagonally before serving.

Kale and Quinoa Stuffed Bell Peppers:

Ingredients:

- 4 bell peppers, halved and seeds removed
- 1 cup quinoa, cooked
- 2 cups kale, finely chopped
- 1 can (15 oz) black beans, drained and rinsed
- 1 cup corn kernels (fresh, frozen, or canned)
- 1 cup cherry tomatoes, diced
- 1/2 cup red onion, finely chopped
- 2 cloves garlic, minced
- 1 teaspoon ground cumin
- 1 teaspoon chili powder
- Salt and pepper to taste
- 1 cup shredded cheese (cheddar, mozzarella, or a blend)
- Olive oil for drizzling

Instructions:

1. Preheat the oven to 375°F (190°C).
2. Place the bell pepper halves in a baking dish.
3. In a large bowl, combine cooked quinoa, chopped kale, black beans, corn, cherry tomatoes, red onion, minced garlic, ground cumin, chili powder, salt, and pepper. Mix well.
4. Spoon the quinoa mixture into each bell pepper half, pressing it down gently.
5. Drizzle a little olive oil over each stuffed pepper.
6. Cover the baking dish with aluminum foil and bake for 25-30 minutes, or until the peppers are tender.
7. Remove the foil, sprinkle shredded cheese over the top of each stuffed pepper, and return to the oven for an additional 5-7 minutes until the cheese is melted and bubbly.
8. Remove from the oven and let it cool slightly before serving.

Caprese Salad with Balsamic Glaze:

Ingredients:

- 4 large tomatoes, sliced
- 8 ounces (about 225g) fresh mozzarella cheese, sliced
- Fresh basil leaves
- 1/4 cup extra-virgin olive oil
- 2 tablespoons balsamic glaze
- Salt and pepper to taste

Instructions:

1. Arrange the tomato slices and fresh mozzarella slices alternately on a serving platter.
2. Tuck fresh basil leaves between the tomato and mozzarella slices.
3. Drizzle extra-virgin olive oil over the arranged slices.
4. Generously drizzle balsamic glaze over the salad.
5. Sprinkle salt and pepper to taste.
6. Optional: Garnish with additional fresh basil leaves.
7. Serve immediately as a refreshing Caprese Salad.

Veggie Stir-Fry with Tofu:

Ingredients:

- 1 block extra-firm tofu, pressed and cubed
- 2 tablespoons soy sauce
- 1 tablespoon sesame oil
- 1 tablespoon vegetable oil
- 1 bell pepper, thinly sliced
- 1 carrot, julienned
- 1 broccoli crown, cut into florets
- 1 zucchini, sliced
- 2 cups snap peas, ends trimmed

- 3 cloves garlic, minced
- 1 tablespoon ginger, grated
- 2 tablespoons hoisin sauce
- 1 tablespoon rice vinegar
- Cooked brown rice or noodles for serving
- Sesame seeds and green onions for garnish (optional)

Instructions:

1. In a bowl, toss the cubed tofu with soy sauce and sesame oil. Let it marinate for 15-20 minutes.
2. Heat vegetable oil in a large skillet or wok over medium-high heat.
3. Add the marinated tofu and cook until golden brown on all sides. Remove from the skillet and set aside.
4. In the same skillet, add a bit more oil if needed. Stir-fry the bell pepper, carrot, broccoli, zucchini, and snap peas until they are tender-crisp.
5. Add minced garlic and grated ginger to the vegetables, stir-frying for an additional 1-2 minutes.
6. Return the cooked tofu to the skillet.
7. In a small bowl, mix hoisin sauce and rice vinegar. Pour the sauce over the tofu and vegetables. Toss everything together until well coated and heated through.
8. Serve the veggie stir-fry over cooked brown rice or noodles.
9. Garnish with sesame seeds and green onions if desired.

Chickpea and Spinach Quesadilla:

Ingredients:

- 1 can (15 oz) chickpeas, drained and rinsed
- 2 cups fresh spinach leaves
- 1/2 red onion, finely chopped
- 1 teaspoon ground cumin
- 1 teaspoon paprika

- Salt and pepper to taste
- 4 large whole-grain tortillas
- 1 1/2 cups shredded cheese (cheddar, mozzarella, or a blend)
- Olive oil for cooking
- Greek yogurt or salsa for serving (optional)

Instructions:

1. In a skillet, heat olive oil over medium heat. Add chopped red onion and sauté until softened.
2. Add chickpeas to the skillet and season with ground cumin, paprika, salt, and pepper. Cook for 3-5 minutes until chickpeas are heated through and coated with the spices.
3. Add fresh spinach leaves to the skillet and cook until wilted. Remove from heat and set aside.
4. Place a tortilla on a clean surface. Spread a layer of the chickpea and spinach mixture on half of the tortilla.
5. Sprinkle a generous amount of shredded cheese over the chickpea mixture.
6. Fold the tortilla in half, creating a quesadilla.
7. Repeat the process with the remaining tortillas.
8. In a large skillet, heat a bit of olive oil over medium heat. Cook each quesadilla for 2-3 minutes on each side or until the tortilla is crispy and the cheese is melted.
9. Repeat until all quesadillas are cooked.
10. Slice the quesadillas into wedges and serve with Greek yogurt or salsa if desired.

Shrimp and Mango Salad:

Ingredients:

- 1 pound (about 450g) shrimp, peeled and deveined
- 2 ripe mangoes, peeled, pitted, and diced
- 1 cucumber, diced
- 1 red bell pepper, diced

- 1/4 red onion, finely chopped
- 1/4 cup fresh cilantro, chopped
- Juice of 2 limes
- 2 tablespoons olive oil
- Salt and pepper to taste
- Mixed salad greens for serving

Instructions:

1. In a large pot of boiling water, cook the shrimp for 2-3 minutes or until they turn pink and opaque. Drain and let them cool.
2. In a large bowl, combine the cooked shrimp, diced mangoes, cucumber, red bell pepper, red onion, and cilantro.
3. In a small bowl, whisk together lime juice, olive oil, salt, and pepper to create the dressing.
4. Pour the dressing over the shrimp and mango mixture. Toss gently to coat.
5. Refrigerate the salad for at least 30 minutes to allow the flavors to meld.
6. Serve the Shrimp and Mango Salad over a bed of mixed salad greens.

Sweet Potato and Lentil Soup:

Ingredients:

- 1 cup dried green or brown lentils, rinsed and drained
- 2 large sweet potatoes, peeled and diced
- 1 onion, chopped
- 2 carrots, peeled and sliced
- 2 celery stalks, chopped
- 3 cloves garlic, minced
- 1 teaspoon ground cumin
- 1 teaspoon ground coriander
- 1/2 teaspoon smoked paprika
- 6 cups vegetable broth

- 1 can (14 oz) diced tomatoes
- 2 tablespoons tomato paste
- Salt and pepper to taste
- 2 tablespoons olive oil
- Fresh parsley for garnish (optional)

Instructions:

1. In a large pot, heat olive oil over medium heat. Add chopped onion, carrots, celery, and garlic. Sauté until the vegetables are softened.
2. Add ground cumin, ground coriander, and smoked paprika to the pot. Stir to coat the vegetables with the spices.
3. Add sweet potatoes, lentils, vegetable broth, diced tomatoes, and tomato paste to the pot. Season with salt and pepper to taste.
4. Bring the soup to a boil, then reduce the heat and let it simmer for 25-30 minutes or until the sweet potatoes and lentils are tender.
5. Adjust the seasoning if needed and let the soup rest for a few minutes before serving.
6. Garnish with fresh parsley if desired.

Grilled Chicken Caesar Salad:

Ingredients:

- 2 boneless, skinless chicken breasts
- Salt and black pepper to taste
- 1 tablespoon olive oil
- 1 teaspoon dried oregano
- 1 teaspoon garlic powder
- Romaine lettuce, washed and chopped
- 1 cup cherry tomatoes, halved
- 1/2 cup croutons
- 1/2 cup freshly grated Parmesan cheese

For Caesar Dressing:

- 1/3 cup mayonnaise
- 2 tablespoons grated Parmesan cheese
- 2 tablespoons lemon juice
- 1 tablespoon Dijon mustard
- 1 clove garlic, minced
- Salt and black pepper to taste

Instructions:

1. Preheat the grill or grill pan to medium-high heat.
2. Season the chicken breasts with salt, black pepper, dried oregano, and garlic powder. Drizzle with olive oil.
3. Grill the chicken for 6-8 minutes per side or until fully cooked. Let it rest for a few minutes before slicing.
4. In a small bowl, whisk together all the Caesar dressing ingredients until well combined.
5. In a large bowl, toss the chopped romaine lettuce with cherry tomatoes and croutons.
6. Add the sliced grilled chicken on top of the salad.
7. Drizzle the Caesar dressing over the salad and chicken.
8. Sprinkle freshly grated Parmesan cheese on top.
9. Toss the salad gently to coat everything with the dressing.
10. Serve immediately, garnished with additional Parmesan cheese if desired.

Dinner Recipes:

Baked Lemon Herb Cod:

Ingredients:

- 4 cod fillets
- 2 tablespoons olive oil

- 2 tablespoons fresh lemon juice
- 2 teaspoons lemon zest
- 2 cloves garlic, minced
- 1 teaspoon dried thyme
- 1 teaspoon dried rosemary
- Salt and black pepper to taste
- Lemon slices for garnish
- Fresh parsley for garnish

Instructions:

1. Preheat the oven to 400°F (200°C). Line a baking sheet with parchment paper.
2. Place the cod fillets on the prepared baking sheet.
3. In a small bowl, whisk together olive oil, fresh lemon juice, lemon zest, minced garlic, dried thyme, dried rosemary, salt, and black pepper.
4. Pour the lemon herb mixture over the cod fillets, ensuring they are evenly coated.
5. Place a few lemon slices on top of each fillet for additional flavor.
6. Bake in the preheated oven for 12-15 minutes or until the cod is opaque and flakes easily with a fork.
7. Remove from the oven and garnish with fresh parsley.
8. Serve the Baked Lemon Herb Cod with your favorite side dishes.

Quinoa and Black Bean Stuffed Peppers

Ingredients:

- 4 large bell peppers, halved and seeds removed
- 1 cup quinoa, rinsed
- 2 cups vegetable broth or water
- 1 can (15 oz) black beans, drained and rinsed
- 1 cup corn kernels (fresh, frozen, or canned)
- 1 cup diced tomatoes
- 1 cup diced red onion

- 2 cloves garlic, minced
- 1 teaspoon ground cumin
- 1 teaspoon chili powder
- Salt and pepper to taste
- 1 cup shredded cheese (cheddar, Monterey Jack, or a blend)
- Fresh cilantro **or parsley for garnish**

Instructions:

1. Preheat the oven to 375°F (190°C).
2. In a saucepan, combine quinoa and vegetable broth (or water). Bring to a boil, then reduce heat, cover, and simmer for 15-20 minutes or until the quinoa is cooked and liquid is absorbed.
3. In a large bowl, mix the cooked quinoa, black beans, corn, diced tomatoes, red onion, minced garlic, ground cumin, chili powder, salt, and pepper.
4. Place the bell pepper halves in a baking dish.
5. Spoon the quinoa and black bean mixture into each bell pepper half.
6. Top each stuffed pepper with shredded cheese.
7. Cover the baking dish with aluminum foil and bake for 25-30 minutes or until the peppers are tender.
8. Remove the foil and bake for an additional 5-7 minutes until the cheese is melted and bubbly.
9. Garnish with fresh cilantro or parsley before serving.

Teriyaki Tofu Stir-Fry:

Ingredients:

- 1 block extra-firm tofu, pressed and cubed
- 1/2 cup teriyaki sauce
- 2 tablespoons soy sauce
- 1 tablespoon sesame oil
- 1 tablespoon vegetable oil

- 1 tablespoon fresh ginger, grated
- 2 cloves garlic, minced
- 1 bell pepper, thinly sliced
- 1 carrot, julienned
- 1 cup broccoli florets
- 1 cup snap peas, ends trimmed
- Cooked brown rice or noodles for serving
- Sesame seeds and green onions for garnish (optional)

Instructions:

1. In a bowl, toss the cubed tofu with teriyaki sauce and soy sauce. Let it marinate for 15-20 minutes.
2. In a large skillet or wok, heat vegetable oil over medium-high heat.
3. Add marinated tofu to the skillet and cook until it turns golden brown on all sides. Remove from the skillet and set aside.
4. In the same skillet, add sesame oil and sauté grated ginger and minced garlic until fragrant.
5. Add bell pepper, julienned carrot, broccoli florets, and snap peas to the skillet. Stir-fry for 3-5 minutes or until the vegetables are tender-crisp.
6. Return the cooked tofu to the skillet and toss everything together.
7. Serve the Teriyaki Tofu Stir-Fry over cooked brown rice or noodles.

Zucchini Noodles with Pesto:

Ingredients:

- 4 medium-sized zucchinis, spiralized into noodles
- 1 cup fresh basil leaves
- 1/2 cup grated Parmesan cheese
- 1/3 cup pine nuts
- 2 cloves garlic, minced
- 1/2 cup extra-virgin olive oil

- Salt and black pepper to taste
- Cherry tomatoes for garnish (optional)

Instructions:

1. In a food processor, combine basil, Parmesan cheese, pine nuts, and minced garlic.
2. Pulse the ingredients until coarsely chopped.
3. With the food processor running, slowly pour in the olive oil until the pesto reaches a smooth consistency.
4. Season the pesto with salt and black pepper to taste. Adjust the seasoning if needed.
5. In a large skillet, heat a bit of olive oil over medium heat.
6. Add the zucchini noodles to the skillet and sauté for 2-3 minutes until just tender.
7. Add the prepared pesto to the zucchini noodles and toss until the noodles are evenly coated.
8. Cook for an additional 2 minutes, stirring occasionally to heat the pesto.
9. Remove from heat and garnish with cherry tomatoes if desired.

Mushroom and Spinach Stuffed Chicken Breast:

Ingredients:
- 4 boneless, skinless chicken breasts
- Salt and black pepper to taste
- 1 tablespoon olive oil
- 8 oz mushrooms, finely chopped
- 2 cups fresh spinach, chopped
- 2 cloves garlic, minced
- 1/2 cup shredded mozzarella cheese
- 1/4 cup grated Parmesan cheese
- 1 teaspoon dried thyme
- 1 teaspoon dried rosemary
- 1/2 cup chicken broth
- 1 tablespoon butter
- Fresh parsley for garnish

Instructions:

1. Preheat the oven to 375°F (190°C).
2. Season each chicken breast with salt and black pepper.
3. In a skillet, heat olive oil over medium heat.
4. Sauté chopped mushrooms until they release their moisture and become golden brown.
5. Add minced garlic and chopped spinach to the skillet. Cook until the spinach is wilted.
6. Remove the skillet from heat and stir in mozzarella cheese, Parmesan cheese, dried thyme, and dried rosemary.
7. Make a horizontal slit in each chicken breast to create a pocket.
8. Stuff each chicken breast with the mushroom and spinach mixture.
9. Secure the openings with toothpicks if needed.
10. In the same skillet, heat chicken broth and butter over medium heat until the butter is melted.
11. Place the stuffed chicken breasts in the skillet and sear each side for 2-3 minutes or until golden brown.
12. Transfer the skillet to the preheated oven and bake for 20-25 minutes or until the chicken is cooked through.
13. Garnish with fresh parsley before serving.

Eggplant and Chickpea Curry:

Ingredients:

- 1 large eggplant, diced
- 1 can (15 oz) chickpeas, drained and rinsed
- 1 onion, finely chopped
- 2 tomatoes, diced
- 3 cloves garlic, minced
- 1 tablespoon fresh ginger, grated
- 2 tablespoons curry powder
- 1 teaspoon ground cumin
- 1 teaspoon ground coriander
- 1/2 teaspoon turmeric powder
- 1/2 teaspoon chili powder (adjust to taste)

- 1 can (14 oz) coconut milk
- 1 cup vegetable broth
- Salt and black pepper to taste
- 2 tablespoons olive oil
- Fresh cilantro for garnish
- Cooked rice or naan for serving

Instructions:

1. In a large skillet or pot, heat olive oil over medium heat.
2. Add chopped onion and sauté until softened.
3. Stir in minced garlic and grated ginger, cooking for an additional minute.
4. Add curry powder, ground cumin, ground coriander, turmeric powder, and chili powder to the skillet. Stir well to coat the onion mixture with the spices.
5. Add diced eggplant and chickpeas to the skillet, stirring to combine.
6. Pour in diced tomatoes, coconut milk, and vegetable broth. Season with salt and black pepper to taste.
7. Bring the mixture to a simmer and let it cook for 20-25 minutes or until the eggplant is tender and the flavors are well combined.
8. Adjust seasoning if needed and garnish with fresh cilantro.
9. Serve the Eggplant and Chickpea Curry over cooked rice or with naan.

Cauliflower and Chickpea Tacos:

Ingredients:

- 1 head cauliflower, cut into small florets
- 1 can (15 oz) chickpeas, drained and rinsed
- 2 tablespoons olive oil
- 1 teaspoon ground cumin
- 1 teaspoon smoked paprika
- 1/2 teaspoon chili powder
- Salt and black pepper to taste

- 8 small corn or flour tortillas
- Toppings: Shredded lettuce, diced tomatoes, sliced red onion, avocado slices, cilantro, lime wedges
- Optional: Greek yogurt or salsa for drizzling

Instructions:

1. Preheat the oven to 400°F (200°C).
2. In a large bowl, toss cauliflower florets and chickpeas with olive oil, ground cumin, smoked paprika, chili powder, salt, and black pepper until evenly coated.
3. Spread the cauliflower and chickpea mixture on a baking sheet in a single layer.
4. Roast in the preheated oven for 20-25 minutes or until the cauliflower is golden brown and chickpeas are crispy, stirring halfway through.
5. Warm the tortillas in a dry skillet or microwave.
6. Assemble the tacos by placing a spoonful of the roasted cauliflower and chickpea mixture onto each tortilla.
7. Top with shredded lettuce, diced tomatoes, sliced red onion, avocado slices, and cilantro.
8. Drizzle with Greek yogurt or salsa if desired.
9. Serve with lime wedges on the side.

Salmon and Asparagus Foil Packets:

Ingredients:

- 4 salmon fillets
- 1 bunch asparagus, trimmed
- 4 tablespoons olive oil
- 4 cloves garlic, minced
- 2 tablespoons lemon juice
- 1 teaspoon dried dill
- Salt and black pepper to taste
- Lemon slices for garnish

- Fresh parsley for garnish

Instructions:

1. Preheat the oven to 400°F (200°C).
2. Cut four large pieces of aluminum foil, each large enough to wrap around a salmon fillet and asparagus.
3. Place a salmon fillet in the center of each piece of foil.
4. Arrange asparagus around each salmon fillet.
5. In a small bowl, whisk together olive oil, minced garlic, lemon juice, dried dill, salt, and black pepper.
6. Drizzle the olive oil mixture evenly over each salmon fillet and asparagus.
7. Fold the foil over the salmon and asparagus, sealing the edges to create packets.
8. Place the foil packets on a baking sheet and bake in the preheated oven for 15-20 minutes or until the salmon is cooked through and flakes easily.
9. Carefully open the foil packets, garnish with lemon slices and fresh parsley.
10. Serve the Salmon and Asparagus Foil Packets directly from the foil.

Mango Salsa Chicken:

Ingredients:

- 4 boneless, skinless chicken breasts
- Salt and black pepper to taste
- 1 tablespoon olive oil
- 1 teaspoon cumin
- 1 teaspoon paprika
- 1/2 teaspoon garlic powder
- 1/2 teaspoon onion powder
- 1/2 teaspoon chili powder
- **For Mango Salsa:**
    - 2 ripe mangoes, peeled, pitted, and diced
    - 1/2 red onion, finely chopped

- 1 jalapeño, seeds removed and finely chopped
- 1 red bell pepper, diced
- 1/4 cup fresh cilantro, chopped
- Juice of 2 limes
- Salt to taste

Instructions:

1. Preheat the oven to 375°F (190°C).
2. Season each chicken breast with salt, black pepper, cumin, paprika, garlic powder, onion powder, and chili powder.
3. In an oven-safe skillet, heat olive oil over medium-high heat.
4. Sear the seasoned chicken breasts for 2-3 minutes on each side until golden brown.
5. Transfer the skillet to the preheated oven and bake for 20-25 minutes or until the chicken is cooked through.
6. While the chicken is baking, prepare the Mango Salsa. In a bowl, combine diced mangoes, chopped red onion, jalapeño, red bell pepper, cilantro, lime juice, and salt. Mix well.
7. Once the chicken is done, top each breast with a generous spoonful of Mango Salsa.
8. Serve the Mango Salsa Chicken over rice or with your favorite side dishes.

Vegetarian Lentil Lasagna:

Ingredients:

- 9 lasagna noodles, cooked according to package instructions
- 2 cups cooked green or brown lentils
- 1 tablespoon olive oil
- 1 onion, finely chopped
- 3 cloves garlic, minced
- 1 zucchini, grated
- 1 carrot, grated
- 1 bell pepper, finely chopped
- 1 can (14 oz) crushed tomatoes

- 1 can (6 oz) tomato paste
- 1 teaspoon dried oregano
- 1 teaspoon dried basil
- 1/2 teaspoon dried thyme
- Salt and black pepper to taste
- 2 cups ricotta cheese
- 2 cups shredded mozzarella cheese
- 1/2 cup grated Parmesan cheese
- Fresh basil for garnish (optional)

Instructions:

1. Preheat the oven to 375°F (190°C).
2. In a large skillet, heat olive oil over medium heat. Add chopped onion and minced garlic, sautéing until softened.
3. Add grated zucchini, grated carrot, and chopped bell pepper to the skillet. Cook for 5-7 minutes or until the vegetables are tender.
4. Stir in crushed tomatoes, tomato paste, dried oregano, dried basil, dried thyme, salt, and black pepper. Simmer for 10-15 minutes, allowing the flavors to meld.
5. In a separate bowl, combine cooked lentils with half of the tomato sauce mixture.
6. In another bowl, mix ricotta cheese with salt and black pepper to taste.
7. Spread a small amount of the remaining tomato sauce on the bottom of a baking dish.
8. Arrange a layer of cooked lasagna noodles over the sauce.
9. Spread half of the lentil mixture over the noodles, followed by half of the ricotta mixture and a sprinkle of mozzarella and Parmesan cheese.
10. Repeat the layers with the remaining noodles, lentil mixture, ricotta mixture, and cheeses.
11. Finish with a layer of noodles topped with the remaining tomato sauce.
12. Sprinkle additional mozzarella and Parmesan cheese on top.
13. Cover the baking dish with aluminum foil and bake in the preheated oven for 30 minutes.
14. Remove the foil and bake for an additional 15-20 minutes or until the cheese is melted and bubbly.
15. Let the Vegetarian Lentil Lasagna rest for a few minutes before slicing.
16. Garnish with fresh basil if desired before serving.

Spaghetti Squash Primavera:

Ingredients:

- 1 medium-sized spaghetti squash
- 2 tablespoons olive oil
- 1 onion, thinly sliced
- 2 carrots, julienned
- 1 zucchini, julienned
- 1 yellow bell pepper, thinly sliced
- 2 cloves garlic, minced
- 1 cup cherry tomatoes, halved
- 1/2 cup fresh basil, chopped
- Salt and black pepper to taste
- Grated Parmesan cheese for serving (optional)

Instructions:

1. Preheat the oven to 375°F (190°C).
2. Cut the spaghetti squash in half lengthwise and scoop out the seeds.
3. Place the squash halves, cut side down, on a baking sheet. Bake for 35-45 minutes or until the squash is tender and easily pierced with a fork.
4. While the squash is baking, heat olive oil in a large skillet over medium heat.
5. Add sliced onion, julienned carrots, julienned zucchini, and sliced bell pepper to the skillet. Sauté for 5-7 minutes or until the vegetables are tender-crisp.
6. Add minced garlic and halved cherry tomatoes to the skillet. Cook for an additional 2 minutes.
7. Use a fork to scrape the strands of cooked spaghetti squash into the skillet with the sautéed vegetables.
8. Toss everything together to combine and heat through.
9. Stir in chopped fresh basil. Season with salt and black pepper to taste.
10. Serve the Spaghetti Squash Primavera with grated Parmesan cheese on top if desired.

CHAPTER 4: SNACKS AND SIDES

Greek Yogurt and Berries:

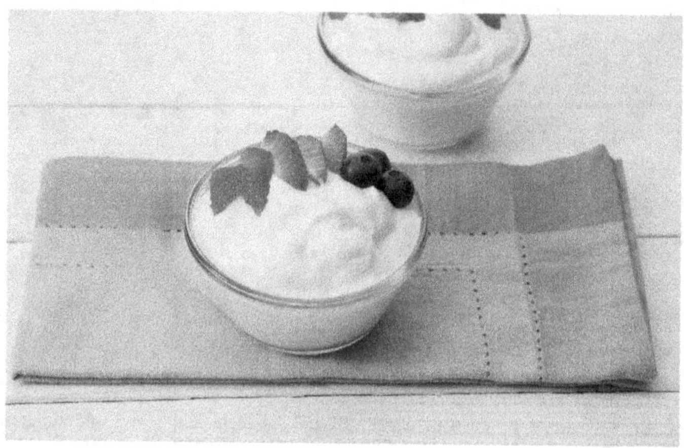

Ingredients:

- 1 cup Greek yogurt
- 1 cup mixed berries (strawberries, blueberries, raspberries, blackberries)
- 1 tablespoon honey or maple syrup (optional)
- 1/4 teaspoon vanilla extract (optional)
- Fresh mint leaves for garnish (optional)

Instructions:

1. In a bowl, spoon out the Greek yogurt.
2. Wash and prepare the mixed berries, then layer them on top of the Greek yogurt.
3. If desired, drizzle honey or maple syrup over the berries for added sweetness.
4. Optionally, add a splash of vanilla extract for extra flavor.
5. Garnish with fresh mint leaves for a refreshing touch.
6. Mix gently just before serving to combine the yogurt and berries.

Guacamole with Veggie Sticks:

Ingredients:

- 3 ripe avocados, peeled and pitted
- 1 small red onion, finely chopped
- 2 tomatoes, diced
- 1/4 cup fresh cilantro, chopped
- 1-2 cloves garlic, minced
- Juice of 1-2 limes
- Salt and pepper to taste
- Carrot sticks, cucumber slices, and bell pepper strips for dipping

Instructions:

1. In a bowl, mash the ripe avocados with a fork until creamy but still a bit chunky.
2. Add finely chopped red onion, diced tomatoes, chopped cilantro, minced garlic, and lime juice to the mashed avocados.
3. Season with salt and pepper to taste.
4. Mix all the ingredients together until well combined.
5. Adjust lime juice, salt, and pepper as needed.
6. Serve the guacamole in a bowl alongside carrot sticks, cucumber slices, and bell pepper strips for dipping.

Trail Mix with Nuts and Seeds:

Ingredients:

- 1 cup almonds
- 1 cup walnuts
- 1/2 cup pumpkin seeds
- 1/2 cup sunflower seeds
- 1/2 cup cashews
- 1/2 cup dried cranberries
- 1/2 cup raisins

- 1/2 cup dark chocolate chips
- 1/2 teaspoon sea salt

Instructions:

1. In a dry skillet over medium heat, toast the almonds, walnuts, pumpkin seeds, sunflower seeds, and cashews for 3-5 minutes, stirring frequently until lightly browned and fragrant. Be careful not to burn them.
2. Allow the toasted nuts and seeds to cool completely.
3. In a large bowl, combine the toasted nuts and seeds with dried cranberries, raisins, dark chocolate chips, and sea salt.
4. Mix everything together until evenly distributed.
5. Store the trail mix in an airtight container for freshness.

Hummus and Whole-Grain Crackers:

Ingredients:

- 1 can (15 oz) chickpeas, drained and rinsed
- 1/4 cup tahini
- 1/4 cup olive oil
- 2 cloves garlic, minced
- Juice of 1 lemon
- 1/2 teaspoon ground cumin
- 1/2 teaspoon paprika
- Salt and pepper to taste
- Whole-grain crackers for serving

Instructions:

1. In a food processor, combine chickpeas, tahini, olive oil, minced garlic, lemon juice, ground cumin, paprika, salt, and pepper.
2. Process the ingredients until smooth and creamy. If needed, add a bit of water to achieve your desired consistency.
3. Taste and adjust the seasoning as necessary.

4. Transfer the hummus to a serving bowl.

5. Serve the hummus with whole-grain crackers for dipping.

Apple Slices with Almond Butter:

Ingredients:

- 2 apples, cored and sliced
- 1/4 cup almond butter
- 1 tablespoon honey (optional)
- 1/2 teaspoon cinnamon (optional)
- Sliced almonds for garnish (optional)

Instructions:

1. Arrange the apple slices on a serving plate.

2. In a small microwave-safe bowl, warm the almond butter for a few seconds until it becomes easily spreadable.

3. Drizzle almond butter over the apple slices or use a knife to spread it on each slice.

4. Optional: Drizzle honey over the almond butter for added sweetness and sprinkle cinnamon on top for extra flavor.

5. Garnish with sliced almonds if desired.

Roasted Chickpeas:

Ingredients:

- 2 cans (15 oz each) chickpeas, drained and rinsed
- 2 tablespoons olive oil
- 1 teaspoon ground cumin
- 1 teaspoon paprika
- 1/2 teaspoon garlic powder
- 1/2 teaspoon onion powder
- 1/2 teaspoon cayenne pepper (adjust to taste)
- Salt to taste

Instructions:

1. Preheat the oven to 400°F (200°C).
2. Rinse and drain the chickpeas. Pat them dry with a paper towel to remove excess moisture.
3. In a bowl, toss the chickpeas with olive oil, ground cumin, paprika, garlic powder, onion powder, cayenne pepper, and salt until evenly coated.
4. Spread the chickpeas in a single layer on a baking sheet lined with parchment paper.
5. Bake in the preheated oven for 25-30 minutes or until the chickpeas are golden brown and crispy, shaking the pan halfway through for even roasting.
6. Remove from the oven and let the roasted chickpeas cool slightly before serving.

Edamame Pods:

Ingredients:

- 2 cups fresh or frozen edamame pods
- 1 tablespoon olive oil
- 1-2 cloves garlic, minced
- Sea salt to taste

Instructions:

1. If using frozen edamame, thaw them according to the package instructions.
2. In a pot of boiling water, cook the edamame pods for 3-5 minutes or until they are tender.
3. Drain the edamame and pat them dry with a paper towel.
4. In a skillet, heat olive oil over medium heat.
5. Add minced garlic to the skillet and sauté for 1-2 minutes until fragrant.
6. Add the cooked edamame pods to the skillet and stir to coat them in the garlic-infused oil.
7. Sauté the edamame for an additional 2-3 minutes, allowing them to slightly crisp up.

8. Sprinkle sea salt over the edamame pods, tossing to ensure even seasoning.

9. Remove from heat and serve immediately.

Greek Yogurt Parfait with Granola:

Ingredients:

- 1 cup Greek yogurt
- 1 cup granola
- 1 cup mixed berries (strawberries, blueberries, raspberries)
- Honey for drizzling (optional)

Instructions:

1. In a glass or bowl, layer half of the Greek yogurt at the bottom.
2. Add a layer of half the granola over the yogurt.
3. Scatter half of the mixed berries on top of the granola.
4. Repeat the layers with the remaining Greek yogurt, granola, and berries.
5. Drizzle honey over the top if desired.
6. Serve the Greek Yogurt Parfait immediately and enjoy!

Cottage Cheese with Pineapple:

Ingredients:

- 1 cup cottage cheese
- 1 cup fresh pineapple chunks (or canned pineapple tidbits, drained)
- Honey for drizzling (optional)
- Mint leaves for garnish (optional)

Instructions:

1. In a bowl, scoop out the cottage cheese.
2. Add fresh pineapple chunks or drained canned pineapple tidbits on top of the cottage cheese.
3. Optional: Drizzle honey over the cottage cheese and pineapple for added sweetness.

4. Garnish with fresh mint leaves if desired.

5. Serve the Cottage Cheese with Pineapple immediately and enjoy!

Dark Chocolate and Almonds:

Ingredients:

- 1 cup dark chocolate chips or chunks
- 1 cup whole almonds

Instructions:

1. In a microwave-safe bowl, melt the dark chocolate chips in 20-30 second intervals, stirring in between until fully melted.

2. Add whole almonds to the melted chocolate, stirring to coat them evenly.

3. Using a fork or spoon, lift the chocolate-coated almonds one by one, letting excess chocolate drip off, and place them on a parchment paper-lined tray.

4. Allow the chocolate-covered almonds to cool and harden at room temperature or place them in the refrigerator for faster setting.

5. Once the chocolate is fully hardened, break apart any clusters of almonds.

6. Serve and enjoy these Dark Chocolate and Almonds as a sweet and crunchy treat.

Veggie Sushi Rolls:

Ingredients:

- 2 cups sushi rice, cooked and seasoned with rice vinegar, sugar, and salt
- 10 nori (seaweed) sheets
- 1 cucumber, julienned
- 1 carrot, julienned
- 1 avocado, sliced
- 1/2 cup pickled ginger
- Soy sauce for dipping
- Wasabi and/or sesame seeds for garnish (optional)

Instructions:

1. Place a bamboo sushi rolling mat on a clean surface. Put a sheet of plastic wrap over the mat.
2. Lay a nori sheet, shiny side down, on the plastic wrap-covered bamboo mat.
3. Wet your hands and grab a handful of sushi rice. Spread the rice evenly over the nori, leaving a small border at the top.
4. Arrange julienned cucumber, carrot, and avocado slices horizontally in the center of the rice.
5. Lift the edge of the bamboo mat closest to you and roll it over the ingredients, using firm but gentle pressure.
6. Continue rolling until you reach the small border at the top. Wet the border slightly and seal the edge.
7. Using a sharp knife, moisten with water to prevent sticking, slice the roll into bite-sized pieces.
8. Repeat the process with the remaining nori sheets and ingredients.
9. Serve the Veggie Sushi Rolls with pickled ginger, soy sauce, and optional wasabi or sesame seeds.

Side Dishes:

Quinoa and Vegetable Salad:

Ingredients:
- 1 cup quinoa, rinsed
- 2 cups water or vegetable broth
- 1 cucumber, diced
- 1 bell pepper (any color), diced
- 1 cup cherry tomatoes, halved
- 1/2 red onion, finely chopped
- 1/4 cup fresh parsley, chopped
- 1/4 cup feta cheese, crumbled (optional)

- 2 tablespoons olive oil
- 1 tablespoon red wine vinegar
- 1 teaspoon Dijon mustard
- Salt and black pepper to taste
- Lemon wedges for serving (optional)

Instructions:

1. In a saucepan, combine quinoa and water or vegetable broth. Bring to a boil, then reduce heat, cover, and simmer for 15-20 minutes or until quinoa is cooked and liquid is absorbed. Fluff with a fork and let it cool.
2. In a large bowl, combine cooled quinoa, diced cucumber, diced bell pepper, halved cherry tomatoes, chopped red onion, and fresh parsley.
3. In a small bowl, whisk together olive oil, red wine vinegar, Dijon mustard, salt, and black pepper.
4. Pour the dressing over the quinoa and vegetable mixture, tossing to coat evenly.
5. If using, sprinkle crumbled feta cheese over the salad and gently mix.
6. Refrigerate the Quinoa and Vegetable Salad for at least 30 minutes before serving to let the flavors meld.
7. Serve chilled, and optionally, garnish with lemon wedges.

Roasted Sweet Potato Wedges:

Ingredients:

- 2 large sweet potatoes, scrubbed and cut into wedges
- 2 tablespoons olive oil
- 1 teaspoon paprika
- 1 teaspoon garlic powder
- 1 teaspoon onion powder
- 1/2 teaspoon cayenne pepper (optional, for extra heat)
- Salt and black pepper to taste
- Fresh parsley for garnish (optional)

Instructions:

1. Preheat the oven to 425°F (220°C) and line a baking sheet with parchment paper.
2. In a large bowl, toss sweet potato wedges with olive oil, paprika, garlic powder, onion powder, cayenne pepper (if using), salt, and black pepper until evenly coated.
3. Arrange the seasoned sweet potato wedges in a single layer on the prepared baking sheet.
4. Roast in the preheated oven for 25-30 minutes, flipping halfway through, or until the wedges are golden brown and tender.
5. Remove from the oven and let them cool slightly.
6. Optional: Garnish with fresh parsley before serving.

Cauliflower Mash:

Ingredients:

- 1 large head cauliflower, cut into florets
- 2 cloves garlic, minced
- 2 tablespoons unsalted butter or olive oil
- 1/4 cup milk (dairy or plant-based)
- Salt and black pepper to taste
- Chopped fresh chives or parsley for garnish (optional)

Instructions:

1. Steam or boil the cauliflower florets until very tender, about 10-15 minutes.
2. Drain the cauliflower well to remove excess moisture.
3. In a food processor or blender, combine the steamed cauliflower, minced garlic, butter or olive oil, and milk.
4. Blend until smooth and creamy. You may need to scrape down the sides of the processor or blender to ensure even blending.
5. Season the cauliflower mash with salt and black pepper to taste. Adjust the seasoning as needed.

6. Transfer the cauliflower mash to a serving dish.

7. Garnish with chopped fresh chives or parsley if desired.

Steamed Broccoli with Lemon:

Ingredients:

- 1 bunch fresh broccoli, cut into florets
- 1 tablespoon olive oil
- 1-2 tablespoons fresh lemon juice
- Zest of 1 lemon
- Salt and black pepper to taste

Instructions:

1. Steam the broccoli florets until they are crisp-tender, about 5-7 minutes.
2. In a small bowl, whisk together olive oil, fresh lemon juice, and lemon zest.
3. Transfer the steamed broccoli to a serving dish.
4. Drizzle the lemon and olive oil mixture over the broccoli.
5. Season with salt and black pepper to taste.
6. Toss the broccoli gently to coat it with the lemon-infused dressing.
7. Serve the Steamed Broccoli with Lemon immediately.

Grilled Asparagus with Parmesan:

Ingredients:

- **1 bunch fresh** asparagus, woody ends trimmed
- 2 tablespoons olive oil
- 1/4 cup grated Parmesan cheese
- Salt and black pepper to taste
- Lemon wedges for serving (optional)

Instructions:

1. Preheat a grill or grill pan over medium-high heat.
2. Toss the trimmed asparagus with olive oil, ensuring they are well-coated.

3. Grill the asparagus for 3-5 minutes, turning occasionally, until they are tender with a slight char.

4. Remove the grilled asparagus from the heat and place them on a serving platter.

5. Sprinkle grated Parmesan cheese over the hot asparagus, allowing it to melt slightly.

6. Season with salt and black pepper to taste.

7. Optional: Serve with lemon wedges for an extra burst of freshness.

Mango Avocado Salsa:

Ingredients:

- 1 ripe mango, peeled, pitted, and diced
- 1 ripe avocado, peeled, pitted, and diced
- 1/2 red onion, finely chopped
- 1 jalapeño, seeds removed and finely chopped
- 1/4 cup fresh cilantro, chopped
- Juice of 2 limes
- Salt and black pepper to taste

Instructions:

1. In a bowl, combine diced mango, diced avocado, chopped red onion, chopped jalapeño, and chopped cilantro.

2. Squeeze the juice of two limes over the ingredients.

3. Gently toss the salsa until all the ingredients are well combined.

4. Season with salt and black pepper to taste.

5. Refrigerate the Mango Avocado Salsa for at least 30 minutes to let the flavors meld.

6. Serve chilled as a topping for grilled chicken, fish, tacos, or as a refreshing dip with tortilla chips.

Cucumber Tomato Salad:

Ingredients:

- 2 large cucumbers, sliced
- 2 cups cherry tomatoes, halved
- 1/2 red onion, thinly sliced
- 1/4 cup fresh parsley, chopped
- 2 tablespoons olive oil
- 2 tablespoons red wine vinegar
- 1 teaspoon Dijon mustard
- Salt and black pepper to taste
- Feta cheese for garnish (optional)

Instructions:

1. In a large bowl, combine sliced cucumbers, halved cherry tomatoes, thinly sliced red onion, and chopped fresh parsley.
2. In a small bowl, whisk together olive oil, red wine vinegar, Dijon mustard, salt, and black pepper.
3. Pour the dressing over the cucumber and tomato mixture, tossing gently to coat all the ingredients.
4. Optional: Crumble feta cheese over the salad for added creaminess and saltiness.
5. Refrigerate the Cucumber Tomato Salad for at least 15-30 minutes before serving to let the flavors meld.

Quinoa Stuffed Mushrooms:

Ingredients:

- 1 cup quinoa, cooked according to package instructions
- 16-20 large mushrooms, cleaned and stems removed
- 1 tablespoon olive oil
- 1 small onion, finely chopped
- 2 cloves garlic, minced

- 1 cup spinach, chopped
- 1/2 cup feta cheese, crumbled
- 1/4 cup grated Parmesan cheese
- 1 teaspoon dried oregano
- Salt and black pepper to taste
- Fresh parsley for garnish (optional)

Instructions:

1. Preheat the oven to 375°F (190°C).
2. In a skillet, heat olive oil over medium heat. Add chopped onion and minced garlic, sautéing until softened.
3. Add chopped spinach to the skillet and cook until wilted.
4. In a bowl, combine cooked quinoa, sautéed onion, garlic, and spinach, crumbled feta cheese, grated Parmesan cheese, dried oregano, salt, and black pepper. Mix well.
5. Stuff each mushroom cap with the quinoa mixture, pressing down gently to pack it.
6. Arrange the stuffed mushrooms on a baking sheet.
7. Bake in the preheated oven for 20-25 minutes or until the mushrooms are tender and the filling is golden brown.
8. Optional: Garnish with fresh parsley before serving.

Brown Rice Pilaf with Almonds:

Ingredients:

- 1 cup brown rice
- 2 cups vegetable or chicken broth
- 2 tablespoons olive oil or butter
- 1/2 cup slivered almonds
- 1 small onion, finely chopped
- 2 cloves garlic, minced

- 1/4 cup fresh parsley, chopped
- Salt and black pepper to taste

Instructions:

1. Rinse the brown rice under cold water.
2. In a saucepan, heat olive oil or butter over medium heat.
3. Add chopped onion and minced garlic, sautéing until the onion is translucent.
4. Add brown rice to the saucepan and toast for 2-3 minutes, stirring frequently.
5. Pour in the vegetable or chicken broth, bring to a boil, then reduce the heat to low. Cover and simmer for the recommended time on the rice package or until the rice is cooked and liquid is absorbed.
6. While the rice is cooking, in a separate skillet, toast the slivered almonds over medium heat until they are golden brown and fragrant. Be cautious not to burn them.
7. Once the rice is cooked, fluff it with a fork and fold in the toasted almonds and chopped fresh parsley.
8. Season the Brown Rice Pilaf with Almonds with salt and black pepper to taste.
9. Serve the pilaf as a side dish or as a bed for your favorite protein.

Sauteed Spinach with Garlic:

Ingredients:

- 1 bunch fresh spinach, washed and trimmed
- 2 tablespoons olive oil
- 3 cloves garlic, minced
- Salt and black pepper to taste
- Lemon wedges for serving (optional)

Instructions:

1. Heat olive oil in a large skillet over medium heat.
2. Add minced garlic to the skillet and sauté for about 30 seconds until fragrant but not browned.

3. Add the fresh spinach to the skillet in batches, tossing with tongs until wilted.

4. Continue adding batches of spinach until all the leaves are wilted, usually within 2-3 minutes.

5. Season the sautéed spinach with salt and black pepper to taste.

6. Optional: Squeeze fresh lemon juice over the spinach for added brightness.

7. Remove from heat and serve immediately.

Baked Brussels Sprouts with Balsamic Glaze:

Ingredients:

- 1 pound Brussels sprouts, trimmed and halved
- 2 tablespoons olive oil
- Salt and black pepper to taste
- 2 tablespoons balsamic glaze

Instructions:

1. Preheat the oven to 400°F (200°C) and line a baking sheet with parchment paper.

2. In a bowl, toss Brussels sprouts with olive oil, salt, and black pepper until well coated.

3. Spread the Brussels sprouts in a single layer on the prepared baking sheet.

4. Roast in the preheated oven for 20-25 minutes, or until the Brussels sprouts are golden brown and crispy on the edges.

5. While the Brussels sprouts are baking, warm the balsamic glaze in a small saucepan over low heat or in the microwave.

6. Once the Brussels sprouts are done, transfer them to a serving dish and drizzle with balsamic glaze.

7. Toss gently to coat the Brussels sprouts in the glaze.

8. Serve the Baked Brussels Sprouts with Balsamic Glaze as a tasty side dish.

CHAPTER 5: VEGETARIAN AND VEGAN

Eggplant Parmesan:

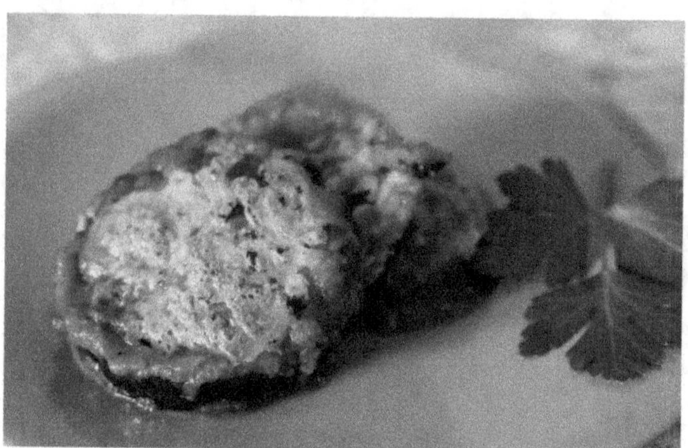

Ingredients:

- 2 large eggplants, sliced into 1/2-inch rounds
- 2 cups gluten-free breadcrumbs
- 1 cup grated parmesan cheese (use a dairy-free alternative if needed)
- 2 cups tomato sauce (look for low-sugar options)
- 1 teaspoon dried oregano
- 1 teaspoon dried basil
- 1/2 teaspoon garlic powder
- Salt and pepper to taste
- Olive oil for baking

Instructions:

1. Preheat your oven to 400°F (200°C).
2. Sprinkle salt over the eggplant slices and let them sit for about 15 minutes to draw out excess moisture. Pat them dry with a paper towel.

3. In a bowl, mix the gluten-free breadcrumbs with grated parmesan cheese, dried oregano, dried basil, garlic powder, salt, and pepper.

4. Dip each eggplant slice into the breadcrumb mixture, ensuring they are well coated on both sides.

5. Place the coated eggplant slices on a baking sheet lined with parchment paper.

6. Bake in the preheated oven for about 20-25 minutes or until the eggplant is tender and the coating is golden brown.

7. In a separate bowl, mix the tomato sauce with additional herbs and seasonings if desired.

8. Once the eggplant slices are done baking, remove them from the oven and reduce the oven temperature to 350°F (175°C).

9. In a baking dish, layer the baked eggplant slices with tomato sauce. Repeat the layers until all the ingredients are used, finishing with a layer of tomato sauce on top.

10. Bake in the 350°F (175°C) oven for an additional 20-25 minutes or until the dish is heated through and bubbly.

11. Allow it to cool for a few minutes before serving.

Vegetarian Chili:

Ingredients:

- 2 tablespoons olive oil
- 1 large onion, chopped
- 3 cloves garlic, minced
- 1 bell pepper, diced (any color)
- 1 zucchini, diced
- 1 carrot, diced
- 1 can (15 oz) black beans, drained and rinsed
- 1 can (15 oz) kidney beans, drained and rinsed
- 1 can (15 oz) pinto beans, drained and rinsed

- 1 can (28 oz) crushed tomatoes
- 1 cup corn kernels (fresh or frozen)
- 1 tablespoon chili powder
- 1 teaspoon cumin
- 1 teaspoon paprika
- 1/2 teaspoon oregano
- Salt and pepper to taste
- 2 cups vegetable broth
- Optional toppings: shredded cheese, chopped green onions, cilantro, sour cream

Instructions:

1. In a large pot, heat olive oil over medium heat. Add chopped onions and minced garlic, sauté until softened.
2. Add diced bell pepper, zucchini, and carrot to the pot. Cook for about 5 minutes until the vegetables are slightly tender.
3. Stir in chili powder, cumin, paprika, oregano, salt, and pepper. Cook for an additional 2 minutes to toast the spices.
4. Add drained and rinsed black beans, kidney beans, pinto beans, crushed tomatoes, corn, and vegetable broth. Stir well to combine.
5. Bring the chili to a boil, then reduce the heat to low. Cover and simmer for at least 30 minutes, allowing the flavors to meld. Stir occasionally.
6. Taste and adjust seasonings as needed. If you prefer a thicker consistency, simmer for a bit longer.
7. Serve hot, and top with shredded cheese, chopped green onions, cilantro, or a dollop of sour cream if desired.

Mushroom and Spinach Stuffed Peppers:

Ingredients:

- 4 large bell peppers, halved and seeds removed
- 2 tablespoons olive oil

- 1 onion, finely chopped
- 2 cloves garlic, minced
- 8 oz mushrooms, finely chopped
- 4 cups fresh spinach, chopped
- 1 cup cooked quinoa or rice
- 1 cup shredded mozzarella or your favorite cheese
- 1 teaspoon dried oregano
- Salt and pepper to taste
- 1 can (15 oz) diced tomatoes, drained (optional, for topping)
- Fresh parsley for garnish (optional)

Instructions:

1. Preheat your oven to 375°F (190°C).
2. Place the halved bell peppers in a baking dish, cut side up.
3. In a large skillet, heat olive oil over medium heat. Add chopped onions and garlic, sauté until softened.
4. Add chopped mushrooms to the skillet and cook until they release their moisture and become golden brown.
5. Stir in chopped spinach and cook until wilted. Season with salt, pepper, and dried oregano.
6. In a large bowl, combine the mushroom and spinach mixture with cooked quinoa or rice.
7. Fill each bell pepper half with the mushroom and spinach mixture, pressing it down gently.
8. Top each stuffed pepper with shredded mozzarella cheese.
9. Bake in the preheated oven for 25-30 minutes or until the peppers are tender and the cheese is melted and bubbly.
10. If desired, top each stuffed pepper with diced tomatoes and fresh parsley before serving.

Vegetarian Buddha Bowl:

Ingredients:

For the Base:

- 2 cups cooked quinoa or brown rice
- 1 cup kale, stems removed and chopped
- 1 cup roasted sweet potatoes, cubed
- 1 cup cherry tomatoes, halved
- 1 avocado, sliced

For the Protein:

- 1 can (15 oz) chickpeas, drained and rinsed
- 1 tablespoon olive oil
- 1 teaspoon smoked paprika
- Salt and pepper to taste

For the Dressing:

- 3 tablespoons tahini
- 2 tablespoons lemon juice
- 2 tablespoons water
- 1 clove garlic, minced
- Salt and pepper to taste

Optional Garnish:

- Sesame seeds
- Chopped cilantro or parsley

Instructions:

1. Preheat the oven to 400°F (200°C).
2. In a bowl, toss the chickpeas with olive oil, smoked paprika, salt, and pepper. Spread them on a baking sheet and roast for about 20-25 minutes or until crispy, shaking the pan occasionally.
3. In a large skillet, sauté kale with a bit of olive oil until wilted. Season with salt and pepper.

4. Assemble the bowls by dividing quinoa or brown rice among serving bowls. Arrange roasted sweet potatoes, cherry tomatoes, sautéed kale, avocado slices, and roasted chickpeas on top.

5. In a small bowl, whisk together tahini, lemon juice, water, minced garlic, salt, and pepper to make the dressing.

6. Drizzle the dressing over the Buddha bowls.

7. Garnish with sesame seeds and chopped cilantro or parsley if desired.

8. Serve immediately and enjoy your nutritious Vegetarian Buddha Bowl!

Caprese Grilled Cheese Sandwich:

Ingredients:

- 4 slices of your favorite bread (sourdough works well)
- 1-2 tablespoons unsalted butter, softened
- 1-2 large tomatoes, sliced
- 8 oz fresh mozzarella, sliced
- Fresh basil leaves
- Balsamic glaze (store-bought or homemade)
- Salt and pepper to taste

Instructions:

1. Heat a skillet or griddle over medium heat.

2. Butter one side of each slice of bread.

3. On the non-buttered side of two slices, layer fresh mozzarella slices, tomato slices, and fresh basil leaves. Season with a pinch of salt and pepper.

4. Drizzle a bit of balsamic glaze over the fillings.

5. Top each sandwich with the remaining slices of bread, buttered side facing out.

6. Place the sandwiches on the heated skillet or griddle. Cook until the bread is golden brown and the cheese is melted, about 3-4 minutes per side.

7. Press the sandwiches down with a spatula while cooking to help the ingredients meld together.

8. Once the sandwiches are golden brown on both sides and the cheese is gooey, remove them from the skillet.

9. Allow the sandwiches to cool for a minute before slicing them in half.

10. Serve your Caprese Grilled Cheese Sandwiches warm and enjoy the delicious combination of mozzarella, tomatoes, and basil!

Vegetarian Sushi Rolls:

Ingredients:

For the Sushi Rice:

- 2 cups sushi rice
- 2 1/2 cups water
- 1/3 cup rice vinegar
- 3 tablespoons sugar
- 1 teaspoon salt

For the Vegetarian Sushi Rolls:

- Nori sheets (seaweed)
- Sushi rice (cooled to room temperature)
- Avocado, thinly sliced
- Cucumber, julienned
- Carrot, julienned
- Bell pepper, thinly sliced
- Cream cheese, sliced (optional)
- Soy sauce and pickled ginger for serving

Instructions:

1. Rinse the sushi rice under cold water until the water runs clear. Cook the rice with water according to the package instructions.

2. While the rice is cooking, in a small saucepan, combine rice vinegar, sugar, and salt. Heat over low heat until the sugar and salt dissolve. Allow the mixture to cool.

3. Once the rice is cooked, transfer it to a large bowl. Gradually add the vinegar mixture, folding it into the rice. Let the rice cool to room temperature.

4. Place a bamboo sushi rolling mat on a flat surface. Put a sheet of plastic wrap on top of the mat.

5. Lay a sheet of nori, shiny side down, on the plastic wrap.

6. Wet your hands to prevent the rice from sticking and spread a thin layer of sushi rice over the nori, leaving a small border at the top.

7. Arrange your desired fillings (avocado, cucumber, carrot, bell pepper, and cream cheese if using) horizontally on the lower third of the rice-covered nori.

8. Lift the edge of the bamboo mat closest to you, and begin rolling the nori over the fillings. Use the mat to shape and tighten the roll.

9. Once the roll is complete, wet the exposed border of the nori to seal the edge.

10. Use a sharp knife to slice the roll into bite-sized pieces.

11. Repeat the process with the remaining nori sheets and fillings.

12. Serve the vegetarian sushi rolls with soy sauce and pickled ginger.

Pesto Zoodles:

Ingredients:

- 4 medium zucchini, spiralized into zoodles
- 1 cup fresh basil leaves, packed
- 1/2 cup grated Parmesan cheese
- 1/3 cup pine nuts
- 2 cloves garlic, peeled
- 1/2 cup extra-virgin olive oil
- Salt and pepper to taste
- Cherry tomatoes for garnish (optional)

Instructions:

1. Prepare the Zoodles:

o   Use a spiralizer to turn the zucchini into zoodles. If you don't have a spiralizer, you can use a vegetable peeler to create thin strips.

2. Make the Pesto:

o   In a food processor, combine basil, Parmesan cheese, pine nuts, and garlic. Pulse until finely chopped.

o   With the food processor running, slowly drizzle in the olive oil until the pesto reaches your desired consistency.

o   Season with salt and pepper to taste.

3. Combine Zoodles and Pesto:

o   In a large pan, heat a bit of olive oil over medium heat.

o   Add the zoodles and cook for 2-3 minutes until they are just tender but still have a slight crunch.

4. Add Pesto:

o   Pour the prepared pesto over the zoodles in the pan.

o   Toss the zoodles in the pesto until they are well coated. Cook for an additional 1-2 minutes.

5. Serve:

o   Transfer the pesto-coated zoodles to serving plates.

o   Optionally, garnish with cherry tomatoes and extra Parmesan cheese.

Spinach and Feta Stuffed Portobello Mushrooms:

Ingredients:

- 4 large portobello mushrooms, stems removed
- 2 tablespoons olive oil
- 1 small onion, finely chopped
- 2 cloves garlic, minced
- 4 cups fresh spinach, chopped
- 1/2 cup feta cheese, crumbled
- 1/4 cup grated Parmesan cheese

- Salt and pepper to taste
- 1/2 teaspoon dried oregano
- 1/2 teaspoon dried thyme
- 1/4 cup breadcrumbs (optional, for topping)
- Fresh parsley for garnish (optional)

Instructions:

1. Preheat the Oven:
   - Preheat your oven to 375°F (190°C).
2. Prepare the Portobello Mushrooms:
   - Clean the portobello mushrooms and remove the stems. Place them on a baking sheet lined with parchment paper.
3. Prepare the Filling:
   - In a large skillet, heat olive oil over medium heat. Add chopped onions and garlic, sauté until softened.
   - Add chopped spinach to the skillet and cook until wilted.
   - Remove the skillet from heat and stir in crumbled feta, grated Parmesan, dried oregano, dried thyme, salt, and pepper. Mix until well combined.
4. Stuff the Mushrooms:
   - Spoon the spinach and feta mixture into each portobello mushroom cap, pressing it down gently.
5. Optional Topping:
   - If desired, sprinkle breadcrumbs on top of each stuffed mushroom for a crispy topping.
6. Bake:
   - Bake in the preheated oven for 20-25 minutes or until the mushrooms are tender and the filling is heated through.
7. Garnish and Serve:
   - Garnish with fresh parsley if desired.
   - Serve the Spinach and Feta Stuffed Portobello Mushrooms warm.

Vegetarian Tacos with Black Beans:

Ingredients:

- 1 can (15 oz) black beans, drained and rinsed
- 1 cup corn kernels (fresh or frozen)
- 1 bell pepper, diced
- 1 onion, finely chopped
- 2 cloves garlic, minced
- 1 teaspoon cumin powder
- 1 teaspoon chili powder
- 1/2 teaspoon smoked paprika
- Salt and pepper to taste
- 1 tablespoon olive oil
- 8 small whole wheat or corn tortillas
- Toppings: Avocado slices, salsa, shredded lettuce, and cilantro

Instructions:

1. In a pan, heat olive oil over medium heat. Add chopped onions, garlic, and bell pepper. Sauté until vegetables are tender.
2. Add black beans, corn, cumin powder, chili powder, smoked paprika, salt, and pepper. Cook for 5-7 minutes, allowing flavors to meld.
3. Warm tortillas according to package instructions or lightly toast them.
4. Spoon the black bean mixture onto each tortilla.
5. Top with avocado slices, salsa, shredded lettuce, and cilantro.
6. Fold the tortillas and serve immediately.

Sweet Potato and Black Bean Quesadillas:

Ingredients:

- 2 medium-sized sweet potatoes, peeled and diced
- 1 can (15 oz) black beans, drained and rinsed
- 1 red onion, finely chopped

- 2 cloves garlic, minced
- 1 teaspoon ground cumin
- 1 teaspoon chili powder
- Salt and pepper to taste
- 4 large whole wheat or corn tortillas
- 1 1/2 cups shredded cheese (cheddar, Monterey Jack, or a blend)
- Olive oil for cooking
- Optional toppings: Avocado slices, salsa, sour cream, and cilantro

Instructions:

1. Boil or steam the diced sweet potatoes until they are tender. Drain and set aside.
2. In a pan, heat olive oil over medium heat. Add chopped red onion and garlic. Sauté until softened.
3. Add the cooked sweet potatoes, black beans, ground cumin, chili powder, salt, and pepper to the pan. Stir well and cook for an additional 3-5 minutes.
4. In a separate skillet, heat a bit of olive oil over medium heat. Place a tortilla in the skillet.
5. Sprinkle a layer of shredded cheese on one half of the tortilla. Spoon some of the sweet potato and black bean mixture over the cheese.
6. Fold the tortilla in half, pressing gently with a spatula. Cook until the cheese is melted and the tortilla is golden brown, then flip and cook the other side.
7. Repeat the process for the remaining tortillas.
8. Once cooked, slice the quesadillas into wedges and serve with optional toppings like avocado slices, salsa, sour cream, and cilantro.

Quinoa and Roasted Vegetable Salad:

Ingredients:

- 1 cup quinoa, rinsed and drained
- 2 cups mixed vegetables (e.g., cherry tomatoes, bell peppers, zucchini, and red onion), chopped

- 2 tablespoons olive oil
- 1 teaspoon dried oregano
- Salt and pepper to taste
- 1/4 cup feta cheese, crumbled (optional)
- 1/4 cup fresh parsley, chopped

Dressing:

- 3 tablespoons olive oil
- 2 tablespoons balsamic vinegar
- 1 teaspoon Dijon mustard
- 1 clove garlic, minced
- Salt and pepper to taste

Instructions:

1. Preheat the oven to 400°F (200°C).
2. In a saucepan, combine quinoa with 2 cups of water. Bring to a boil, then reduce heat, cover, and simmer for 15 minutes or until quinoa is cooked and water is absorbed. Fluff with a fork and let it cool.
3. Toss the chopped vegetables with olive oil, dried oregano, salt, and pepper. Spread them evenly on a baking sheet.
4. Roast the vegetables in the preheated oven for 20-25 minutes or until they are tender and slightly caramelized. Stir halfway through cooking.
5. In a large bowl, combine the cooked quinoa and roasted vegetables.
6. In a small bowl, whisk together the dressing ingredients: olive oil, balsamic vinegar, Dijon mustard, minced garlic, salt, and pepper.
7. Pour the dressing over the quinoa and vegetables, tossing gently to coat.
8. Sprinkle with crumbled feta cheese and chopped fresh parsley.
9. Chill the salad in the refrigerator for at least 30 minutes before serving to enhance flavors.

Vegan Chickpea Curry:

Ingredients:

- 2 cans (15 oz each) chickpeas, drained and rinsed
- 1 onion, finely chopped
- 3 cloves garlic, minced
- 1 thumb-sized piece of ginger, grated
- 1 can (14 oz) diced tomatoes
- 1 can (14 oz) coconut milk
- 1 cup vegetable broth
- 2 tablespoons curry powder
- 1 teaspoon ground cumin
- 1 teaspoon ground coriander
- 1/2 teaspoon turmeric
- 1/4 teaspoon cayenne pepper (optional for extra heat)
- Salt and pepper to taste
- 2 cups spinach or kale, chopped
- Fresh cilantro for garnish
- Cooked rice or naan for serving

Instructions:

1. In a large pan, sauté the chopped onion in a bit of oil over medium heat until translucent.
2. Add minced garlic and grated ginger, cooking for an additional minute until fragrant.
3. Stir in the curry powder, ground cumin, ground coriander, turmeric, and cayenne pepper (if using). Cook for another minute to toast the spices.
4. Pour in the diced tomatoes (with their juices), coconut milk, and vegetable broth. Stir well to combine.

5. Add the drained chickpeas to the mixture. Season with salt and pepper. Bring to a simmer and let it cook for 15-20 minutes, allowing the flavors to meld.

6. Add the chopped spinach or kale to the curry, letting it wilt into the mixture.

7. Taste and adjust the seasoning if necessary. Simmer for an additional 5 minutes.

8. Serve the vegan chickpea curry over cooked rice or with naan bread.

9. Garnish with fresh cilantro before serving.

Vegan Lentil Loaf:

Ingredients:

- 1 cup dry green or brown lentils, rinsed and drained
- 3 cups vegetable broth or water
- 1 tablespoon ground flaxseed mixed with 3 tablespoons water (flax egg)
- 1 onion, finely chopped
- 2 cloves garlic, minced
- 1 carrot, grated
- 1 celery stalk, finely chopped
- 1 cup breadcrumbs (whole wheat or gluten-free)
- 1/2 cup rolled oats
- 1/4 cup tomato paste
- 2 tablespoons soy sauce or tamari
- 1 teaspoon dried thyme
- 1 teaspoon dried rosemary
- 1/2 teaspoon smoked paprika
- Salt and pepper to taste
- Olive oil for greasing

Glaze:

- 1/4 cup ketchup
- 1 tablespoon maple syrup or agave nectar
- 1 tablespoon balsamic vinegar

Instructions:

1. Preheat the oven to 375°F (190°C) and grease a loaf pan with olive oil.

2. In a saucepan, combine lentils and vegetable broth. Bring to a boil, then reduce heat and simmer for 25-30 minutes or until lentils are tender. Drain any excess liquid.

3. In a small bowl, prepare the flax egg by mixing ground flaxseed with water. Let it sit for 5 minutes to thicken.

4. In a large mixing bowl, mash half of the cooked lentils. Add in the flax egg, chopped onion, minced garlic, grated carrot, chopped celery, breadcrumbs, rolled oats, tomato paste, soy sauce, dried thyme, dried rosemary, smoked paprika, salt, and pepper. Mix until well combined.

5. Fold in the remaining whole lentils.

6. Transfer the mixture into the greased loaf pan, pressing it down evenly.

7. In a separate bowl, whisk together the ingredients for the glaze: ketchup, maple syrup or agave nectar, and balsamic vinegar.

8. Spread the glaze over the top of the lentil loaf.

9. Bake in the preheated oven for 40-45 minutes or until the top is golden brown and the loaf is firm.

10. Allow the lentil loaf to cool for a few minutes before slicing and serving.

Vegan Stir-Fried Tofu with Vegetables:

Ingredients:

- 1 block (14 oz) firm tofu, pressed and cubed
- 2 tablespoons soy sauce or tamari
- 1 tablespoon sesame oil
- 1 tablespoon cornstarch
- 2 tablespoons vegetable oil
- 1 bell pepper, thinly sliced
- 1 carrot, julienned

- 1 cup broccoli florets
- 2 cloves garlic, minced
- 1 tablespoon ginger, grated
- 3 green onions, chopped
- 1 tablespoon rice vinegar
- 1 tablespoon maple syrup or agave nectar
- 1 tablespoon sesame seeds (optional)
- Cooked brown rice or noodles for serving

Instructions:

1. In a bowl, combine cubed tofu with soy sauce, sesame oil, and cornstarch. Gently toss to coat the tofu evenly. Allow it to marinate for at least 15 minutes.
2. Heat vegetable oil in a wok or large pan over medium-high heat.
3. Add the marinated tofu cubes to the hot pan. Stir-fry until the tofu is golden brown on all sides. Remove tofu from the pan and set aside.
4. In the same pan, add a bit more oil if needed. Sauté bell pepper, carrot, and broccoli until they are slightly tender but still crisp.
5. Add minced garlic and grated ginger to the vegetables. Stir-fry for an additional minute until fragrant.
6. Return the cooked tofu to the pan with the vegetables.
7. In a small bowl, mix rice vinegar and maple syrup or agave nectar. Pour the mixture over the tofu and vegetables. Toss everything together to combine.
8. Add chopped green onions and continue to stir-fry for another 2-3 minutes.
9. Sprinkle sesame seeds on top if desired.
10. Serve the vegan stir-fried tofu and vegetables over cooked brown rice or noodles.

Vegan Spinach and Artichoke Dip:

Ingredients:

- 1 cup raw cashews, soaked in hot water for 1 hour
- 1 tablespoon olive oil

- 1 onion, finely chopped
- 2 cloves garlic, minced
- 1 can (14 oz) artichoke hearts, drained and chopped
- 1 cup frozen chopped spinach, thawed and squeezed dry
- 1/2 cup nutritional yeast
- 1/4 cup lemon juice
- 1/2 teaspoon garlic powder
- 1/2 teaspoon onion powder
- 1/2 teaspoon smoked paprika
- Salt and pepper to taste
- 1/4 cup vegan mayonnaise
- 1/4 cup unsweetened almond milk (or any plant-based milk)
- 1 cup vegan mozzarella or cheddar cheese, shredded (optional)
- Fresh parsley for garnish
- Sliced baguette, tortilla chips, or vegetable sticks for dipping

Instructions:

1. Preheat the oven to 375°F (190°C).
2. In a high-speed blender or food processor, blend the soaked cashews with 1/2 cup of water until smooth and creamy. Set aside.
3. In a pan, heat olive oil over medium heat. Sauté chopped onion until translucent.
4. Add minced garlic and cook for an additional minute until fragrant.
5. Stir in chopped artichoke hearts and thawed, squeezed dry spinach. Cook for 3-5 minutes until heated through.
6. In a large bowl, combine the blended cashew mixture, nutritional yeast, lemon juice, garlic powder, onion powder, smoked paprika, salt, and pepper.
7. Add the sautéed vegetable mixture to the bowl, followed by vegan mayonnaise and almond milk. Mix until well combined.
8. If using vegan cheese, fold it into the mixture.
9. Transfer the dip to a baking dish and spread it evenly.

10. Bake in the preheated oven for 20-25 minutes, or until the top is golden and the edges are bubbling.

11. Remove from the oven and let it cool for a few minutes before serving.

12. Garnish with fresh parsley and serve the vegan spinach and artichoke dip with sliced baguette, tortilla chips, or vegetable sticks for dipping.

Vegan Stuffed Acorn Squash:

Ingredients:

- 2 acorn squashes, halved and seeds removed
- 1 cup quinoa, rinsed
- 2 cups vegetable broth or water
- 1 tablespoon olive oil
- 1 onion, finely chopped
- 2 cloves garlic, minced
- 1 carrot, diced
- 1 celery stalk, diced
- 1 apple, cored and diced
- 1/2 cup dried cranberries
- 1/2 cup chopped pecans or walnuts (optional)
- 1 teaspoon dried thyme
- 1 teaspoon ground sage
- Salt and pepper to taste
- Fresh parsley for garnish

Instructions:

1. Preheat the oven to 400°F (200°C).

2. Place acorn squash halves cut side down on a baking sheet. Roast in the preheated oven for 25-30 minutes or until the squash is fork-tender.

3. While the squash is roasting, rinse quinoa under cold water. In a saucepan, combine quinoa and vegetable broth or water. Bring to a boil, then reduce heat,

cover, and simmer for 15 minutes or until quinoa is cooked and water is absorbed. Fluff with a fork and set aside.

4. In a large pan, heat olive oil over medium heat. Add chopped onion, garlic, carrot, and celery. Sauté until vegetables are softened.
5. Add diced apple, dried cranberries, chopped nuts (if using), dried thyme, ground sage, salt, and pepper to the pan. Cook for an additional 3-5 minutes.
6. Combine the cooked quinoa with the sautéed vegetable mixture. Adjust seasoning if needed.
7. Once the acorn squash halves are done roasting, flip them over and stuff each half with the quinoa and vegetable mixture.
8. Return the stuffed squash to the oven and bake for an additional 15-20 minutes until the tops are golden.
9. Garnish with fresh parsley before serving.

Vegan Pad Thai:

Ingredients:

- 8 oz rice noodles
- 2 tablespoons vegetable oil
- 1 block (14 oz) firm tofu, pressed and cubed
- 1 cup broccoli florets
- 1 carrot, julienned
- 1 bell pepper, thinly sliced
- 3 green onions, sliced
- 2 cloves garlic, minced
- 1/4 cup roasted peanuts, chopped (for garnish)

Sauce:

- 3 tablespoons soy sauce or tamari
- 2 tablespoons tamarind paste
- 2 tablespoons maple syrup or agave nectar

- 1 tablespoon rice vinegar

- 1 teaspoon Sriracha sauce (adjust to taste)

- 1 tablespoon vegetable oil

Instructions:

1. Cook rice noodles according to package instructions. Drain and set aside.

2. In a small bowl, whisk together the sauce ingredients: soy sauce, tamarind paste, maple syrup or agave nectar, rice vinegar, Sriracha sauce, and vegetable oil. Set aside.

3. Heat vegetable oil in a large wok or pan over medium-high heat.

4. Add cubed tofu and stir-fry until golden brown. Remove tofu from the pan and set aside.

5. In the same pan, add a bit more oil if needed. Sauté minced garlic until fragrant.

6. Add broccoli, julienned carrot, and sliced bell pepper to the pan. Stir-fry for 3-5 minutes until the vegetables are tender-crisp.

7. Push the vegetables to the side of the pan and add the cooked rice noodles. Pour the prepared sauce over the noodles and toss everything together.

8. Add the cooked tofu back into the pan and stir to combine.

9. Stir in sliced green onions and cook for an additional 2 minutes.

10. Taste and adjust the seasoning if needed.

11. Serve the vegan Pad Thai hot, garnished with chopped roasted peanuts.

Vegan BBQ Jackfruit Tacos:

Ingredients:

- 2 cans (20 oz each) young green jackfruit in water or brine, drained and shredded

- 1 tablespoon vegetable oil

- 1 onion, finely chopped

- 2 cloves garlic, minced

- 1/2 cup barbecue sauce (vegan-friendly)

- 1 teaspoon smoked paprika

- 1/2 teaspoon cumin
- 1/2 teaspoon chili powder
- Salt and pepper to taste
- 8 small corn or flour tortillas
- Coleslaw for topping (optional)
- Fresh cilantro for garnish
- Lime wedges for serving

Instructions:

1. In a large pan, heat vegetable oil over medium heat. Add chopped onion and sauté until translucent.
2. Add minced garlic to the pan and cook for an additional minute until fragrant.
3. Add shredded jackfruit to the pan, stirring to combine with the onions and garlic.
4. Sprinkle smoked paprika, cumin, chili powder, salt, and pepper over the jackfruit. Mix well to coat the jackfruit with the spices.
5. Pour the barbecue sauce over the jackfruit mixture. Stir to combine, ensuring the jackfruit is evenly coated in the sauce.
6. Cook the jackfruit mixture over medium heat for 10-15 minutes, stirring occasionally. The jackfruit should absorb the flavors and have a tender, pulled texture.
7. While the jackfruit is cooking, warm the tortillas in a dry skillet or microwave according to package instructions.
8. Once the jackfruit is ready, assemble the tacos by spooning the BBQ jackfruit onto each tortilla.
9. Top with coleslaw if desired, and garnish with fresh cilantro.
10. Serve the vegan BBQ jackfruit tacos with lime wedges on the side.

Vegan Chickpea and Vegetable Curry:

Ingredients:

- 1 tablespoon coconut oil or vegetable oil

- 1 onion, finely chopped
- 3 cloves garlic, minced
- 1 thumb-sized piece of ginger, grated
- 1 bell pepper, diced
- 1 zucchini, diced
- 1 carrot, sliced
- 1 can (15 oz) chickpeas, drained and rinsed
- 1 can (14 oz) diced tomatoes
- 1 can (14 oz) coconut milk
- 2 tablespoons curry powder
- 1 teaspoon ground cumin
- 1/2 teaspoon turmeric
- 1/2 teaspoon coriander
- 1/4 teaspoon cayenne pepper (optional for heat)
- Salt and pepper to taste
- Fresh cilantro for garnish
- Cooked rice or naan for serving

Instructions:

1. In a large pan or pot, heat coconut oil over medium heat. Add chopped onion and sauté until translucent.
2. Add minced garlic and grated ginger, cooking for an additional minute until fragrant.
3. Stir in curry powder, ground cumin, turmeric, coriander, and cayenne pepper (if using). Cook for another minute to toast the spices.
4. Add diced bell pepper, zucchini, and sliced carrot to the pan. Sauté until the vegetables are slightly tender.
5. Pour in diced tomatoes, coconut milk, and drained chickpeas. Season with salt and pepper. Stir well to combine.

6. Bring the curry to a simmer, then reduce heat to low and let it cook for 15-20 minutes, allowing the flavors to meld and the vegetables to fully cook.

7. Taste and adjust seasoning if necessary.

8. Serve the vegan chickpea and vegetable curry over cooked rice or with naan bread.

9. Garnish with fresh cilantro before serving.

Vegan Mediterranean Bowl:

Ingredients:

For the Falafel:

- 1 can (15 oz) chickpeas, drained and rinsed
- 1/2 cup fresh parsley, chopped
- 1/4 cup red onion, finely chopped
- 2 cloves garlic, minced
- 1 teaspoon ground cumin
- 1 teaspoon ground coriander
- Salt and pepper to taste
- 2 tablespoons chickpea flour or all-purpose flour
- 2 tablespoons olive oil for cooking

For the Bowl:

- Cooked quinoa or couscous
- Cherry tomatoes, halved
- Cucumber, diced
- Kalamata olives, pitted and sliced
- Red onion, thinly sliced
- Hummus for dressing
- Fresh parsley for garnish
- Lemon wedges for serving

Instructions:

1. Prepare Falafel:

- In a food processor, combine chickpeas, fresh parsley, red onion, minced garlic, ground cumin, ground coriander, salt, and pepper. Pulse until the mixture is coarsely ground.
  - Transfer the mixture to a bowl and stir in chickpea flour or all-purpose flour.
  - Form the mixture into small patties or balls.
  - Heat olive oil in a pan over medium heat. Cook the falafel until golden brown on both sides, about 3-4 minutes per side. Set aside.

2. Assemble the Bowl:
   - Arrange cooked quinoa or couscous in the base of each bowl.
   - Add cherry tomatoes, diced cucumber, sliced Kalamata olives, and thinly sliced red onion around the quinoa or couscous.

3. Add Falafel:
   - Place the cooked falafel on top of the grains and veggies.

4. Drizzle with Hummus:
   - Drizzle hummus over the bowl for added creaminess and flavor.

5. Garnish:
   - Garnish the bowl with fresh parsley.

6. Serve:
   - Serve the Mediterranean bowl with lemon wedges on the side for an extra burst of freshness.

Vegan Coconut Lentil Soup:

Ingredients:

- 1 cup dry brown or green lentils, rinsed
- 1 tablespoon coconut oil
- 1 onion, finely chopped
- 3 cloves garlic, minced
- 1 thumb-sized piece of ginger, grated

- 1 bell pepper, diced
- 2 carrots, diced
- 1 can (14 oz) diced tomatoes
- 1 can (14 oz) coconut milk
- 4 cups vegetable broth
- 1 teaspoon curry powder
- 1/2 teaspoon ground turmeric
- 1/2 teaspoon ground cumin
- 1/2 teaspoon coriander
- Salt and pepper to taste
- Juice of 1 lime
- Fresh cilantro for garnish
- Cooked rice for serving (optional)

Instructions:

1. In a large pot, heat coconut oil over medium heat. Add chopped onion and sauté until translucent.
2. Add minced garlic and grated ginger, cooking for an additional minute until fragrant.
3. Stir in diced bell pepper and carrots. Sauté for 3-5 minutes until the vegetables start to soften.
4. Add rinsed lentils, diced tomatoes (with their juices), coconut milk, and vegetable broth to the pot.
5. Season with curry powder, ground turmeric, ground cumin, coriander, salt, and pepper. Stir well to combine.
6. Bring the soup to a boil, then reduce heat to low, cover, and simmer for 20-25 minutes or until the lentils are tender.
7. Taste and adjust seasoning if necessary.
8. Just before serving, stir in the lime juice for a burst of freshness.
9. Serve the vegan coconut lentil soup hot, garnished with fresh cilantro.

10. Optionally, serve over cooked rice for a heartier meal.

Vegan Chocolate Avocado Mousse:

Ingredients:

- 2 ripe avocados, peeled and pitted
- 1/2 cup cocoa powder
- 1/2 cup maple syrup or agave nectar
- 1/4 cup coconut milk (or any plant-based milk)
- 1 teaspoon vanilla extract
- Pinch of salt
- Optional toppings: Fresh berries, chopped nuts, or coconut flakes

Instructions:

1. Prepare Avocados:
   - In a food processor or blender, combine the ripe avocados.
2. Add Cocoa Powder:
   - Add cocoa powder to the avocados in the processor.
3. Sweeten It:
   - Pour in maple syrup or agave nectar for sweetness.
4. Blend:
   - Blend the mixture until smooth and creamy, scraping down the sides as needed.
5. Add Liquid:
   - Add coconut milk (or any plant-based milk) gradually while blending to achieve the desired consistency.
6. Season:
   - Add vanilla extract and a pinch of salt. Blend again to incorporate.
7. Taste and Adjust:
   - Taste the mousse and adjust the sweetness or thickness if necessary by adding more sweetener or milk.

8. Chill:
    - Transfer the chocolate avocado mousse to a bowl or individual serving glasses.
    - Chill in the refrigerator for at least 1-2 hours to allow it to set.
9. Serve:
    - Once chilled, serve the vegan chocolate avocado mousse with your choice of toppings such as fresh berries, chopped nuts, or coconut flakes.

CHAPTER 6: FISH AND SEAFOODS

Baked Lemon Herb Salmon:

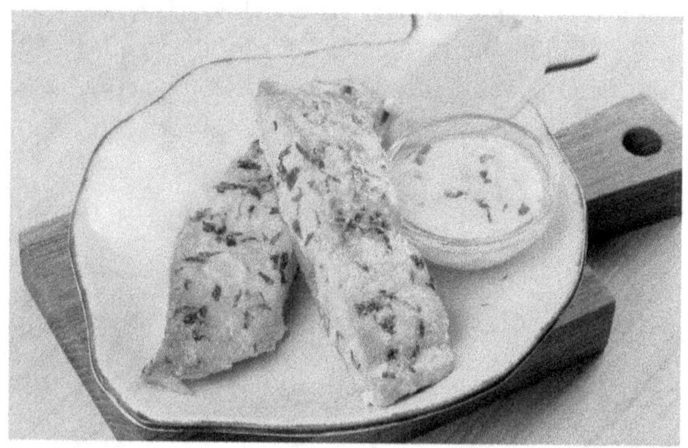

Ingredients:

- 4 salmon fillets
- 2 tablespoons olive oil
- 2 tablespoons lemon juice
- 2 cloves garlic, minced
- 1 teaspoon dried thyme
- 1 teaspoon dried rosemary
- 1 teaspoon dried oregano
- 1/2 teaspoon sea salt
- 1/4 teaspoon black pepper
- Lemon slices for garnish

Instructions:

1. Preheat your oven to 375°F (190°C).

2. In a small bowl, whisk together olive oil, lemon juice, minced garlic, dried thyme, dried rosemary, dried oregano, sea salt, and black pepper.

3. Place the salmon fillets on a baking sheet lined with parchment paper or lightly greased.

4. Brush the salmon fillets evenly with the prepared lemon herb mixture, ensuring they are well coated.

5. Place a few lemon slices on top of each salmon fillet for extra flavor.

6. Bake in the preheated oven for 15-20 minutes or until the salmon flakes easily with a fork.

7. Once done, remove from the oven and let it rest for a couple of minutes before serving.

Grilled Teriyaki Mahi-Mahi:

Ingredients:

- 4 Mahi-Mahi fillets
- 1/2 cup teriyaki sauce
- 2 tablespoons soy sauce
- 2 tablespoons honey
- 1 tablespoon sesame oil
- 2 cloves garlic, minced
- 1 teaspoon ginger, grated
- 1 tablespoon sesame seeds (optional, for garnish)
- Green onions, chopped (optional, for garnish)

Instructions:

1. In a bowl, mix together teriyaki sauce, soy sauce, honey, sesame oil, minced garlic, and grated ginger to create the marinade.

2. Place Mahi-Mahi fillets in a shallow dish or a resealable plastic bag. Pour half of the teriyaki marinade over the fillets, ensuring they are well coated. Reserve the remaining marinade for later use.

3. Marinate the Mahi-Mahi in the refrigerator for at least 30 minutes, allowing the flavors to infuse.

4. Preheat the grill to medium-high heat. Lightly oil the grill grates to prevent sticking.

5. Remove the Mahi-Mahi from the marinade and discard the used marinade.

6. Grill the Mahi-Mahi fillets for about 4-6 minutes per side, or until the fish easily flakes with a fork and has grill marks.

7. Brush the reserved teriyaki marinade over the fillets during the last couple of minutes of grilling for extra flavor.

8. Once done, transfer the grilled Mahi-Mahi to a serving platter.

9. Garnish with sesame seeds and chopped green onions if desired.

Pan-Seared Tilapia with Mango Salsa:

Ingredients:

For Pan-Seared Tilapia:

- 4 tilapia fillets
- 2 tablespoons olive oil
- 1 teaspoon paprika
- 1 teaspoon cumin
- 1/2 teaspoon garlic powder
- Salt and black pepper to taste
- Fresh lime wedges for serving

For Mango Salsa:

- 1 ripe mango, peeled, pitted, and diced
- 1/2 red onion, finely chopped
- 1 red bell pepper, diced
- 1 jalapeño, seeds removed and finely chopped
- 1/4 cup fresh cilantro, chopped
- Juice of 1 lime

- Salt to taste

Instructions:

1. In a small bowl, mix paprika, cumin, garlic powder, salt, and black pepper. Rub the spice mixture evenly over both sides of each tilapia fillet.
2. Heat olive oil in a large skillet over medium-high heat.
3. Place the seasoned tilapia fillets in the skillet and cook for 3-4 minutes per side or until the fish is cooked through and easily flakes with a fork.
4. While the tilapia is cooking, prepare the mango salsa. In a bowl, combine diced mango, red onion, red bell pepper, jalapeño, cilantro, lime juice, and salt. Mix well.
5. Once the tilapia is cooked, transfer the fillets to serving plates.
6. Top each tilapia fillet with a generous spoonful of mango salsa.
7. Serve the pan-seared tilapia with mango salsa alongside fresh lime wedges for added citrus flavor.

Herb-Crusted Cod with Tomato Relish:

Ingredients:

For Herb-Crusted Cod:

- 4 cod fillets
- 2 tablespoons olive oil
- 1 cup breadcrumbs
- 2 tablespoons fresh parsley, finely chopped
- 1 tablespoon fresh dill, finely chopped
- 1 teaspoon dried oregano
- Salt and black pepper to taste
- Lemon wedges for serving

For Tomato Relish:

- 2 cups cherry tomatoes, halved
- 1/4 cup red onion, finely chopped

- 2 tablespoons fresh basil, chiffonade (thin strips)
- 1 tablespoon balsamic vinegar
- 2 tablespoons olive oil
- Salt and black pepper to taste

Instructions:

1. Preheat your oven to 400°F (200°C).
2. In a bowl, combine breadcrumbs, chopped fresh parsley, chopped fresh dill, dried oregano, salt, and black pepper to create the herb crust mixture.
3. Brush each cod fillet with olive oil, ensuring they are well-coated.
4. Press the herb crust mixture onto both sides of each cod fillet, creating an even coating.
5. Place the herb-crusted cod fillets on a baking sheet lined with parchment paper or lightly greased.
6. Bake in the preheated oven for 12-15 minutes or until the cod is cooked through and the crust is golden brown.
7. While the cod is baking, prepare the tomato relish. In a bowl, combine halved cherry tomatoes, finely chopped red onion, chiffonade of fresh basil, balsamic vinegar, olive oil, salt, and black pepper. Toss gently to combine.
8. Once the cod is done baking, transfer the fillets to serving plates.
9. Spoon the tomato relish over the herb-crusted cod fillets.
10. Serve the dish with lemon wedges on the side for added zest.

Coconut Curry Shrimp:

Ingredients:

- 1 pound large shrimp, peeled and deveined
- 2 tablespoons coconut oil
- 1 onion, finely chopped
- 3 cloves garlic, minced
- 1 tablespoon fresh ginger, grated

- 2 tablespoons red curry paste
- 1 can (14 ounces) coconut milk
- 1 cup vegetable broth
- 1 red bell pepper, sliced
- 1 zucchini, sliced
- 1 carrot, julienned
- 1 tablespoon soy sauce
- 1 tablespoon fish sauce
- 1 tablespoon brown sugar
- Juice of 1 lime
- Fresh cilantro, chopped (for garnish)
- Cooked rice for serving

Instructions:

1. In a large skillet or wok, heat coconut oil over medium heat.
2. Add finely chopped onion, minced garlic, and grated ginger. Sauté until the onions are soft and fragrant.
3. Stir in red curry paste and cook for an additional minute to release its flavors.
4. Add coconut milk and vegetable broth to the skillet, stirring to combine.
5. Add the sliced red bell pepper, zucchini, and julienned carrot to the coconut curry mixture. Simmer for 5-7 minutes until the vegetables are tender.
6. Season the shrimp with soy sauce and fish sauce. Add the seasoned shrimp to the skillet and cook for 3-4 minutes until they turn pink and opaque.
7. Stir in brown sugar and lime juice. Adjust seasoning to taste.
8. Once the shrimp are cooked through and the vegetables are tender, remove the skillet from heat.
9. Serve the Coconut Curry Shrimp over cooked rice.
10. Garnish with fresh cilantro and serve immediately.

Cajun-Style Blackened Catfish:

Ingredients:

- 4 catfish fillets
- 2 tablespoons paprika
- 1 tablespoon dried thyme
- 1 tablespoon onion powder
- 1 tablespoon garlic powder
- 1 teaspoon cayenne pepper
- 1 teaspoon black pepper
- 1 teaspoon white pepper
- 1 teaspoon dried oregano
- 1 teaspoon salt
- 4 tablespoons unsalted butter, melted
- Lemon wedges for serving

Instructions:

1. Preheat a cast-iron skillet over medium-high heat.
2. In a bowl, mix together paprika, dried thyme, onion powder, garlic powder, cayenne pepper, black pepper, white pepper, dried oregano, and salt to create the Cajun seasoning.
3. Pat the catfish fillets dry with a paper towel.
4. Brush each catfish fillet with melted butter, ensuring they are well-coated.
5. Sprinkle the Cajun seasoning evenly on both sides of each catfish fillet, pressing the seasoning into the fish.
6. Place the catfish fillets in the preheated cast-iron skillet. Cook for 3-4 minutes on each side or until the fish is blackened and flakes easily with a fork.
7. Remove the skillet from heat and let the catfish rest for a couple of minutes.
8. Serve the Cajun-Style Blackened Catfish with lemon wedges on the side.

Lemon Garlic Butter Trout

Ingredients:

- 4 trout fillets
- 4 tablespoons unsalted butter, melted
- 3 cloves garlic, minced
- Zest of 1 lemon
- Juice of 1 lemon
- 1 tablespoon fresh parsley, chopped
- Salt and black pepper to taste

Instructions:

1. Preheat the oven to 400°F (200°C).
2. Place the trout fillets on a baking sheet lined with parchment paper or lightly greased.
3. In a small bowl, mix together melted butter, minced garlic, lemon zest, lemon juice, chopped fresh parsley, salt, and black pepper to create the lemon garlic butter mixture.
4. Brush each trout fillet with the lemon garlic butter mixture, ensuring they are well-coated on both sides.
5. Bake in the preheated oven for 10-12 minutes or until the trout is cooked through and flakes easily with a fork.
6. While the trout is baking, baste it with the lemon garlic butter mixture every few minutes for added flavor.
7. Once done, remove the trout from the oven and let it rest for a couple of minutes.
8. Serve the Lemon Garlic Butter Trout with additional lemon wedges on the side.

Soy-Ginger Glazed Tuna Steaks:

Ingredients:

- 4 tuna steaks
- 1/4 cup soy sauce

- 2 tablespoons rice vinegar
- 1 tablespoon honey
- 1 tablespoon fresh ginger, grated
- 2 cloves garlic, minced
- 1 tablespoon sesame oil
- 1 tablespoon green onions, chopped (for garnish)
- Sesame seeds (optional, for garnish)

Instructions:

1. In a bowl, whisk together soy sauce, rice vinegar, honey, grated fresh ginger, minced garlic, and sesame oil to create the soy-ginger glaze.
2. Place the tuna steaks in a shallow dish or a resealable plastic bag.
3. Pour half of the soy-ginger glaze over the tuna steaks, ensuring they are well coated. Reserve the remaining glaze for later use.
4. Marinate the tuna steaks in the refrigerator for at least 30 minutes, allowing the flavors to infuse.
5. Preheat a grill or grill pan over medium-high heat.
6. Remove the tuna steaks from the marinade and discard the used marinade.
7. Grill the tuna steaks for 2-3 minutes per side for a medium-rare doneness, or adjust the cooking time based on your preference.
8. While grilling, brush the reserved soy-ginger glaze over the tuna steaks for added flavor.
9. Once done, transfer the grilled tuna steaks to a serving platter.
10. Garnish with chopped green onions and sesame seeds if desired.

Pesto Grilled Swordfish:

Ingredients:

For Swordfish Marinade:

- 4 swordfish steaks
- 1/4 cup olive oil

- 2 tablespoons lemon juice
- 2 cloves garlic, minced
- Salt and black pepper to taste

For Pesto Sauce:

- 2 cups fresh basil leaves, packed
- 1/2 cup grated Parmesan cheese
- 1/3 cup pine nuts
- 2 cloves garlic
- 1/2 cup extra-virgin olive oil
- Salt and black pepper to taste

Instructions:

1. In a bowl, mix together olive oil, lemon juice, minced garlic, salt, and black pepper to create the swordfish marinade.
2. Place the swordfish steaks in a shallow dish or a resealable plastic bag. Pour the marinade over the swordfish, ensuring they are well coated. Marinate in the refrigerator for at least 30 minutes.
3. Meanwhile, prepare the pesto sauce. In a food processor, combine fresh basil, grated Parmesan cheese, pine nuts, garlic, salt, and black pepper. Pulse until finely chopped.
4. With the food processor running, gradually add the olive oil until the pesto reaches a smooth consistency. Adjust seasoning to taste.
5. Preheat a grill or grill pan over medium-high heat.
6. Remove the swordfish steaks from the marinade and discard the used marinade.
7. Grill the swordfish steaks for 3-4 minutes per side or until they are cooked through and have grill marks.
8. During the last minute of grilling, brush each swordfish steak with a generous layer of pesto sauce.
9. Once done, transfer the grilled swordfish steaks to a serving platter.
10. Serve the Pesto Grilled Swordfish with extra pesto on the side for dipping.

Miso Glazed Cod:

Ingredients:

- 4 cod fillets
- 1/4 cup white miso paste
- 2 tablespoons mirin (sweet rice wine)
- 2 tablespoons soy sauce
- 1 tablespoon rice vinegar
- 1 tablespoon honey
- 2 teaspoons sesame oil
- 2 teaspoons fresh ginger, grated
- 2 cloves garlic, minced
- Green onions, chopped (for garnish)
- Sesame seeds (optional, for garnish)

Instructions:

1. In a bowl, whisk together white miso paste, mirin, soy sauce, rice vinegar, honey, sesame oil, grated fresh ginger, and minced garlic to create the miso glaze.
2. Preheat the oven to 400°F (200°C).
3. Place the cod fillets in a baking dish lined with parchment paper or lightly greased.
4. Brush each cod fillet with a generous layer of the miso glaze, ensuring they are well coated on both sides.
5. Bake in the preheated oven for 12-15 minutes or until the cod is cooked through and flakes easily with a fork.
6. While the cod is baking, baste it with the miso glaze every few minutes for added flavor.
7. Once done, remove the cod from the oven and let it rest for a couple of minutes.
8. Transfer the miso glazed cod to serving plates.
9. Garnish with chopped green onions and sesame seeds if desired.

Smoked Paprika and Lime Grilled Sardines:

Ingredients:

- 8 fresh sardines, cleaned and gutted
- 2 tablespoons olive oil
- 2 teaspoons smoked paprika
- Zest of 2 limes
- Juice of 1 lime
- 2 cloves garlic, minced
- Salt and black pepper to taste
- Fresh cilantro, chopped (for garnish)
- Lime wedges (for serving)

Instructions:

1. Preheat a grill or grill pan over medium-high heat.
2. In a bowl, mix together olive oil, smoked paprika, lime zest, lime juice, minced garlic, salt, and black pepper to create the marinade.
3. Pat the sardines dry with a paper towel.
4. Brush each sardine with the smoked paprika and lime marinade, ensuring they are well-coated on both sides.
5. Place the marinated sardines on the preheated grill. Grill for 3-4 minutes per side or until the sardines are cooked through and have grill marks.
6. While grilling, baste the sardines with any remaining marinade for added flavor.
7. Once done, transfer the grilled sardines to a serving platter.
8. Garnish with chopped fresh cilantro and serve with lime wedges on the side.

Seafood Recipes:

Lemon Garlic Butter Shrimp Scampi:

Ingredients:

- 1 pound large shrimp, peeled and deveined

- 8 ounces linguine or spaghetti
- 4 tablespoons unsalted butter
- 4 cloves garlic, minced
- 1/2 cup chicken broth
- Juice of 1 lemon
- Zest of 1 lemon
- 1/4 cup fresh parsley, chopped
- Red pepper flakes (optional, for heat)
- Salt and black pepper to taste
- Grated Parmesan cheese (optional, for serving)

Instructions:

1. Cook the linguine or spaghetti according to the package instructions. Drain and set aside.
2. In a large skillet, melt the butter over medium heat.
3. Add minced garlic to the melted butter and sauté for 1-2 minutes until fragrant.
4. Add the shrimp to the skillet and cook for 2-3 minutes per side or until they turn pink and opaque.
5. Pour in the chicken broth, lemon juice, and lemon zest. Stir to combine.
6. Season the shrimp scampi with salt, black pepper, and red pepper flakes if using. Stir in fresh chopped parsley.
7. Add the cooked linguine or spaghetti to the skillet, tossing to coat the pasta in the lemon garlic butter sauce.
8. Once everything is well combined and heated through, remove from heat.
9. Serve the Lemon Garlic Butter Shrimp Scampi immediately, optionally garnished with grated Parmesan cheese.

Grilled Scallop Skewers with Herb Butter:

Ingredients:

For Scallop Marinade:

- 1 pound large scallops, cleaned and patted dry
- 2 tablespoons olive oil
- 2 tablespoons lemon juice
- 2 cloves garlic, minced
- Salt and black pepper to taste

For Herb Butter:

- 1/2 cup unsalted butter, melted
- 2 tablespoons fresh parsley, finely chopped
- 1 tablespoon fresh dill, finely chopped
- 1 tablespoon fresh chives, finely chopped
- 1 teaspoon lemon zest
- Salt and black pepper to taste

Instructions:

1. In a bowl, mix together olive oil, lemon juice, minced garlic, salt, and black pepper to create the scallop marinade.
2. Place the cleaned scallops in a shallow dish or a resealable plastic bag. Pour the marinade over the scallops, ensuring they are well coated. Marinate in the refrigerator for 15-30 minutes.
3. Preheat a grill or grill pan over medium-high heat.
4. While the grill is heating, prepare the herb butter. In a small bowl, combine melted butter, chopped fresh parsley, chopped fresh dill, chopped fresh chives, lemon zest, salt, and black pepper. Mix well.
5. Thread the marinated scallops onto skewers.
6. Grill the scallop skewers for 2-3 minutes per side or until the scallops are opaque and have grill marks.
7. During the last minute of grilling, brush the scallops generously with the herb butter.
8. Once done, transfer the grilled scallop skewers to a serving platter.
9. Drizzle any remaining herb butter over the top.

10. Serve the Grilled Scallop Skewers with Herb Butter immediately.

Zesty Cilantro Lime Ceviche:

Ingredients:

- 1 pound fresh white fish (such as tilapia or sea bass), diced
- 1/2 cup red onion, finely chopped
- 1 cup cherry tomatoes, halved
- 1 cucumber, diced
- 1 jalapeño, seeds removed and finely chopped
- 1/2 cup fresh cilantro, chopped
- Juice of 4 limes
- Juice of 1 lemon
- Salt and black pepper to taste
- 1 avocado, diced (for garnish)
- Tortilla chips or plantain chips (for serving)

Instructions:

1. In a large bowl, combine diced white fish, finely chopped red onion, halved cherry tomatoes, diced cucumber, finely chopped jalapeño, and chopped fresh cilantro.
2. Squeeze the juice of 4 limes and 1 lemon over the mixture. Stir well to combine.
3. Season the ceviche with salt and black pepper to taste. Mix thoroughly.
4. Cover the bowl with plastic wrap and refrigerate for at least 30 minutes to allow the flavors to meld and the fish to "cook" in the citrus juices. Stir occasionally.
5. Just before serving, gently fold in diced avocado to avoid it from becoming mushy.
6. Serve the Zesty Cilantro Lime Ceviche in individual bowls or on a platter.
7. Garnish with extra cilantro and serve with tortilla chips or plantain chips on the side.

Crab-Stuffed Portobello Mushrooms:

Ingredients:

- 4 large Portobello mushrooms, stems removed and cleaned
- 1 cup lump crabmeat, drained
- 1/4 cup cream cheese, softened
- 2 tablespoons mayonnaise
- 2 tablespoons grated Parmesan cheese
- 1 tablespoon fresh lemon juice
- 1 teaspoon Dijon mustard
- 2 cloves garlic, minced
- 2 green onions, finely chopped
- Salt and black pepper to taste
- 1/4 cup breadcrumbs (optional, for topping)
- Fresh parsley, chopped (for garnish)

Instructions:

1. Preheat the oven to 375°F (190°C).
2. Place the cleaned Portobello mushrooms on a baking sheet.
3. In a bowl, combine lump crabmeat, softened cream cheese, mayonnaise, grated Parmesan cheese, fresh lemon juice, Dijon mustard, minced garlic, chopped green onions, salt, and black pepper. Mix well.
4. Spoon the crab mixture into each Portobello mushroom cap, distributing it evenly.
5. If desired, sprinkle breadcrumbs over the top of each stuffed mushroom for added texture.
6. Bake in the preheated oven for 20-25 minutes or until the mushrooms are tender and the filling is heated through.
7. Once done, remove from the oven and let the stuffed mushrooms rest for a couple of minutes.
8. Garnish with chopped fresh parsley before serving.

Shrimp and Broccoli Stir-Fry:

Ingredients:

- 1 pound large shrimp, peeled and deveined
- 4 cups broccoli florets
- 2 tablespoons soy sauce
- 1 tablespoon oyster sauce
- 1 tablespoon hoisin sauce
- 1 tablespoon sesame oil
- 3 tablespoons vegetable oil, divided
- 3 cloves garlic, minced
- 1 tablespoon fresh ginger, grated
- 1 red bell pepper, thinly sliced
- 1 carrot, julienned
- 4 green onions, sliced
- Cooked rice or noodles (for serving)

Instructions:

1. In a small bowl, mix together soy sauce, oyster sauce, hoisin sauce, and sesame oil to create the stir-fry sauce.
2. Heat 2 tablespoons of vegetable oil in a wok or large skillet over medium-high heat.
3. Add the shrimp and stir-fry for 2-3 minutes or until they turn pink and opaque. Remove the shrimp from the wok and set aside.
4. In the same wok, add the remaining 1 tablespoon of vegetable oil.
5. Add minced garlic and grated ginger to the wok, stirring for about 30 seconds until fragrant.
6. Add broccoli florets, sliced red bell pepper, and julienned carrot to the wok. Stir-fry for 3-4 minutes or until the vegetables are crisp-tender.
7. Return the cooked shrimp to the wok.
8. Pour the stir-fry sauce over the shrimp and vegetables. Toss everything together to coat evenly.
9. Add sliced green onions to the wok and stir-fry for an additional 1-2 minutes.

10. Serve the Shrimp and Broccoli Stir-Fry over cooked rice or noodles.

Garlic Butter Lobster Tails:

Ingredients:

- 4 lobster tails, thawed if frozen
- 1/2 cup unsalted butter, melted
- 4 cloves garlic, minced
- 2 tablespoons fresh parsley, chopped
- 1 tablespoon lemon juice
- Salt and black pepper to taste
- Lemon wedges (for serving)

Instructions:

1. Preheat the oven to 425°F (220°C).
2. Use kitchen shears to cut through the top of the lobster shells lengthwise, stopping at the tail. Carefully lift the lobster meat, leaving it attached at the base, and place it on top of the shells.
3. In a bowl, mix together melted butter, minced garlic, chopped fresh parsley, lemon juice, salt, and black pepper.
4. Brush the garlic butter mixture generously over the exposed lobster meat.
5. Place the prepared lobster tails on a baking sheet lined with parchment paper or in a baking dish.
6. Bake in the preheated oven for 12-15 minutes or until the lobster meat is opaque and cooked through.
7. While baking, baste the lobster tails with the garlic butter mixture every few minutes for added flavor.
8. Once done, remove the lobster tails from the oven and let them rest for a couple of minutes.
9. Serve the Garlic Butter Lobster Tails with lemon wedges on the side.

Coconut Shrimp Curry:

Ingredients:

- 1 pound large shrimp, peeled and deveined
- 2 tablespoons vegetable oil
- 1 onion, finely chopped
- 3 cloves garlic, minced
- 1 tablespoon ginger, grated
- 2 tablespoons red curry paste
- 1 can (14 ounces) coconut milk
- 1 cup chicken or vegetable broth
- 1 red bell pepper, sliced
- 1 zucchini, sliced
- 1 cup snap peas, trimmed
- 1 tablespoon fish sauce
- 1 tablespoon brown sugar
- Juice of 1 lime
- Fresh cilantro, chopped (for garnish)
- Cooked rice (for serving)

Instructions:

1. In a large skillet or wok, heat vegetable oil over medium heat.
2. Add finely chopped onion, minced garlic, and grated ginger. Sauté until the onions are soft and fragrant.
3. Stir in red curry paste and cook for an additional minute to release its flavors.
4. Add coconut milk and chicken or vegetable broth to the skillet, stirring to combine.
5. Add sliced red bell pepper, sliced zucchini, and snap peas to the coconut curry mixture. Simmer for 5-7 minutes until the vegetables are tender.
6. Season the shrimp with fish sauce and add them to the skillet. Cook for 3-4 minutes or until the shrimp are pink and opaque.

7. Stir in brown sugar and lime juice. Adjust seasoning to taste.

8. Once the shrimp are cooked through and the vegetables are tender, remove the skillet from heat.

9. Serve the Coconut Shrimp Curry over cooked rice.

Baked Stuffed Clams:

Ingredients:

- 24 fresh or frozen clam shells
- 2 dozen littleneck clams, scrubbed and steamed
- 1 cup breadcrumbs
- 1/2 cup grated Parmesan cheese
- 1/4 cup fresh parsley, chopped
- 3 cloves garlic, minced
- 2 tablespoons olive oil
- 1 tablespoon lemon juice
- Salt and black pepper to taste
- Lemon wedges (for serving)

Instructions:

1. Preheat the oven to 400°F (200°C).

2. Shuck the steamed littleneck clams and reserve the clam meat. Clean the clam shells thoroughly.

3. In a bowl, combine breadcrumbs, grated Parmesan cheese, chopped fresh parsley, minced garlic, olive oil, lemon juice, salt, and black pepper. Mix well to create the stuffing mixture.

4. Place the cleaned clam shells on a baking sheet lined with parchment paper or in a baking dish.

5. Spoon the stuffing mixture into each clam shell, pressing it down gently.

6. Top each stuffed clam with a piece of the reserved clam meat.

7. Bake in the preheated oven for 12-15 minutes or until the breadcrumbs are golden brown.

8. Once done, remove the baked stuffed clams from the oven and let them cool for a few minutes.

9. Serve the Baked Stuffed Clams with lemon wedges on the side.

Lemon Herb Grilled Octopus:

Ingredients:

- 2 pounds octopus, cleaned
- 1/4 cup olive oil
- Zest of 1 lemon
- Juice of 2 lemons
- 3 cloves garlic, minced
- 2 tablespoons fresh parsley, chopped
- 1 tablespoon fresh oregano, chopped
- Salt and black pepper to taste
- Lemon wedges (for serving)

Instructions:

1. Preheat the grill to medium-high heat.

2. Bring a large pot of water to a boil. Submerge the cleaned octopus in boiling water for about 2-3 minutes to tenderize it.

3. Remove the octopus from the boiling water and let it cool.

4. In a bowl, mix together olive oil, lemon zest, lemon juice, minced garlic, chopped fresh parsley, chopped fresh oregano, salt, and black pepper to create the marinade.

5. Pat the octopus dry with paper towels.

6. Place the octopus on the preheated grill. Grill for 4-5 minutes per side or until the octopus is charred and cooked through.

7. During the last couple of minutes of grilling, brush the octopus with the lemon herb marinade for added flavor.

8. Once done, remove the grilled octopus from the grill and let it rest for a few minutes.

9. Slice the octopus into bite-sized pieces.

10. Serve the Lemon Herb Grilled Octopus with lemon wedges on the side.

Spicy Cajun Crawfish Boil:

Ingredients:

- 5 pounds live crawfish, washed and purged
- 4 quarts water
- 4 lemons, halved
- 1 cup salt
- 1/2 cup Cajun seasoning
- 1/4 cup Old Bay seasoning
- 6 cloves garlic, smashed
- 4 bay leaves
- 1 onion, quartered
- 4 ears of corn, husked and halved
- 1 pound small red potatoes, halved
- 1 pound smoked sausage, sliced
- 4 tablespoons unsalted butter, melted
- 2 teaspoons cayenne pepper (adjust to taste)
- Lemon wedges and chopped fresh parsley (for serving)

Instructions:

1. Fill a large stockpot with 4 quarts of water and place it on high heat.

2. Squeeze the lemon halves into the pot and add the lemon halves themselves.

3. Stir in the salt, Cajun seasoning, Old Bay seasoning, smashed garlic cloves, bay leaves, and quartered onion.

4. Bring the seasoned water to a rolling boil.

5. Add the halved potatoes and sliced smoked sausage to the boiling water. Cook for about 10 minutes.

6. Add the halved corn and continue boiling for an additional 5 minutes.

7. Add the live crawfish to the boiling water and cook for about 3-4 minutes. The crawfish will turn bright red when they are cooked.

8. Turn off the heat and let the crawfish soak in the seasoned water for an additional 15-20 minutes to absorb the flavors.

9. While the crawfish are soaking, prepare the spicy butter sauce. In a small bowl, mix melted butter and cayenne pepper. Adjust the spice level to your liking.

10. Drain the crawfish, potatoes, corn, and sausage, discarding the boiled garlic, bay leaves, and lemon halves.

11. Spread the boiled crawfish, potatoes, corn, and sausage on a large serving platter.

12. Drizzle the spicy butter sauce over the crawfish boil.

13. Serve the Spicy Cajun Crawfish Boil with lemon wedges and chopped fresh parsley on the side.

Sesame Ginger Glazed Mussels:

Ingredients:

- 2 pounds fresh mussels, cleaned and debearded
- 1/4 cup soy sauce
- 2 tablespoons rice vinegar
- 2 tablespoons honey
- 1 tablespoon sesame oil
- 1 tablespoon fresh ginger, grated
- 2 cloves garlic, minced
- 1 teaspoon cornstarch (optional, for thickening)
- 2 tablespoons green onions, thinly sliced (for garnish)
- 1 tablespoon sesame seeds (for garnish)

- Fresh cilantro, chopped (for garnish)
- Cooked rice or crusty bread (for serving)

Instructions:

1. Rinse the fresh mussels under cold running water, scrubbing off any debris. Remove the beards by pulling them away from the shell.
2. In a bowl, whisk together soy sauce, rice vinegar, honey, sesame oil, grated fresh ginger, and minced garlic to create the sesame ginger glaze.
3. Place the cleaned mussels in a large skillet or wide saucepan.
4. Pour the sesame ginger glaze over the mussels.
5. Cover the skillet or saucepan with a lid and cook over medium-high heat for 5-7 minutes, or until the mussels open. Discard any mussels that do not open.
6. If you prefer a thicker sauce, mix a teaspoon of cornstarch with a tablespoon of water and stir it into the sauce. Cook for an additional 1-2 minutes until the sauce thickens slightly.
7. Once the mussels are cooked, transfer them to a serving bowl, pouring the sauce over the top.
8. Garnish with thinly sliced green onions, sesame seeds, and chopped fresh cilantro.
9. Serve the Sesame Ginger Glazed Mussels over cooked rice or with crusty bread on the side.

CHAPTER 7: POULTRY AND MEAT

Herb-Roasted Chicken:

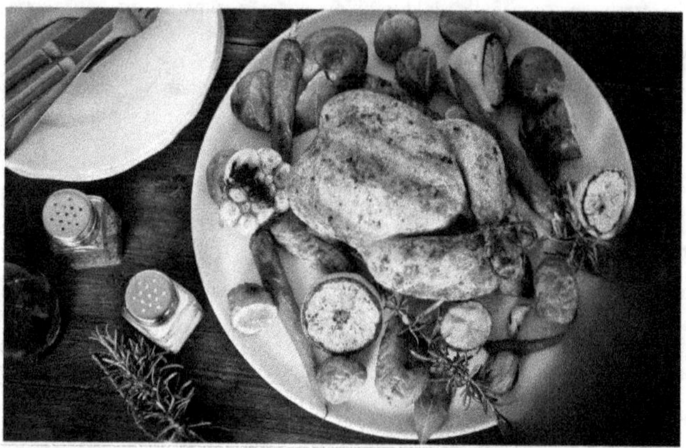

Ingredients:

- 1 whole chicken (about 4-5 pounds), giblets removed
- 2 tablespoons olive oil
- 2 teaspoons dried thyme
- 2 teaspoons dried rosemary
- 2 teaspoons dried sage
- 1 teaspoon dried oregano
- 1 teaspoon dried marjoram
- 1 teaspoon garlic powder
- 1 teaspoon onion powder
- Salt and black pepper to taste
- 1 lemon, halved
- Fresh herbs (thyme, rosemary, sage) for garnish (optional)

Instructions:

1. Preheat the oven to 425°F (220°C).

2. Rinse the whole chicken under cold water and pat it dry with paper towels.

3. In a small bowl, mix together dried thyme, dried rosemary, dried sage, dried oregano, dried marjoram, garlic powder, onion powder, salt, and black pepper.

4. Rub the chicken with olive oil, ensuring it is well-coated.

5. Generously season the chicken with the herb mixture, rubbing it evenly over the entire surface, including the cavity.

6. Place the halved lemon inside the chicken cavity.

7. Tie the chicken legs together with kitchen twine if desired.

8. Transfer the seasoned and stuffed chicken to a roasting pan or baking dish.

9. Roast the chicken in the preheated oven for about 1 hour and 15 minutes or until the internal temperature reaches 165°F (74°C) and the skin is golden and crispy.

10. Once done, remove the herb-roasted chicken from the oven and let it rest for 10-15 minutes before carving.

11. Garnish with fresh herbs if desired.

12. Carve the chicken and serve.

Lemon Garlic Grilled Chicken:

Ingredients:

- 4 boneless, skinless chicken breasts
- 1/4 cup olive oil
- Zest of 2 lemons
- Juice of 2 lemons
- 4 cloves garlic, minced
- 2 teaspoons dried oregano
- 1 teaspoon dried thyme
- Salt and black pepper to taste
- Fresh parsley, chopped (for garnish)

Instructions:

1. In a bowl, whisk together olive oil, lemon zest, lemon juice, minced garlic, dried oregano, dried thyme, salt, and black pepper to create the marinade.
2. Place the chicken breasts in a shallow dish or a resealable plastic bag.
3. Pour the marinade over the chicken, ensuring they are well-coated. Marinate in the refrigerator for at least 30 minutes, or preferably 2-4 hours for more flavor.
4. Preheat the grill to medium-high heat.
5. Remove the chicken from the refrigerator and let it come to room temperature for about 15 minutes.
6. Grill the chicken breasts for 6-8 minutes per side or until they reach an internal temperature of 165°F (74°C) and have nice grill marks.
7. While grilling, baste the chicken with any remaining marinade for added flavor.
8. Once done, transfer the grilled chicken to a serving platter.
9. Garnish with chopped fresh parsley.
10. Serve the Lemon Garlic Grilled Chicken with your favorite sides.

Balsamic Glazed Chicken Thighs:

Ingredients:

- 4 bone-in, skin-on chicken thighs
- 1/4 cup balsamic vinegar
- 2 tablespoons honey
- 2 tablespoons soy sauce
- 2 cloves garlic, minced
- 1 teaspoon Dijon mustard
- 1 teaspoon dried rosemary
- Salt and black pepper to taste
- Fresh parsley, chopped (for garnish)

Instructions:

1. Preheat the oven to 400°F (200°C).

2. Pat the chicken thighs dry with paper towels and season with salt and black pepper.

3. In a small saucepan over medium heat, combine balsamic vinegar, honey, soy sauce, minced garlic, Dijon mustard, and dried rosemary.

4. Bring the mixture to a simmer, stirring occasionally, until it thickens slightly. This usually takes about 5-7 minutes. Remove the saucepan from heat.

5. Place the seasoned chicken thighs in a baking dish.

6. Brush the balsamic glaze over each chicken thigh, ensuring they are well-coated.

7. Bake in the preheated oven for 30-35 minutes or until the chicken thighs are cooked through and the skin is crispy.

8. While baking, baste the chicken thighs with the glaze every 10 minutes for added flavor.

9. Once done, remove the chicken from the oven and let it rest for a couple of minutes.

10. Garnish with chopped fresh parsley.

11. Serve the Balsamic Glazed Chicken Thighs with your favorite side dishes.

Chicken Piccata:

Ingredients:

- 4 boneless, skinless chicken breasts
- Salt and black pepper to taste
- 1/2 cup all-purpose flour, for dredging
- 4 tablespoons unsalted butter
- 4 tablespoons olive oil
- 1/3 cup fresh lemon juice (about 2 lemons)
- 1/2 cup chicken broth
- 1/4 cup capers, drained
- 1/4 cup fresh parsley, chopped (for garnish)
- Lemon slices (for garnish)

Instructions:

1. Season the chicken breasts with salt and black pepper on both sides.
2. Dredge each chicken breast in flour, shaking off excess.
3. In a large skillet, heat 2 tablespoons of butter and 2 tablespoons of olive oil over medium-high heat.
4. Add the chicken breasts to the skillet and cook for about 3-4 minutes per side or until they are golden brown and cooked through. Remove the chicken from the skillet and set aside.
5. In the same skillet, add the remaining 2 tablespoons of butter and 2 tablespoons of olive oil.
6. Stir in fresh lemon juice, chicken broth, and capers. Scrape any browned bits from the bottom of the skillet for added flavor.
7. Bring the sauce to a simmer and cook for 2-3 minutes to allow it to thicken slightly.
8. Return the cooked chicken breasts to the skillet, spooning the sauce over them. Cook for an additional 2 minutes to heat through.
9. Garnish with chopped fresh parsley and lemon slices.
10. Serve the Chicken Piccata over cooked pasta or with your favorite side dishes.

Teriyaki Chicken Skewers:

Ingredients:

- 1.5 pounds boneless, skinless chicken thighs, cut into bite-sized pieces
- 1/2 cup soy sauce
- 1/4 cup mirin (Japanese sweet rice wine)
- 2 tablespoons honey
- 1 tablespoon sake (optional)
- 2 cloves garlic, minced
- 1 teaspoon ginger, grated
- Wooden skewers, soaked in water for 30 minutes

- Sesame seeds (for garnish)
- Green onions, sliced (for garnish)

Instructions:

1. In a bowl, whisk together soy sauce, mirin, honey, sake (if using), minced garlic, and grated ginger to create the teriyaki marinade.
2. Place the bite-sized chicken pieces in a shallow dish or a resealable plastic bag.
3. Pour half of the teriyaki marinade over the chicken, reserving the rest for basting and dipping.
4. Marinate the chicken in the refrigerator for at least 30 minutes, or preferably 2-4 hours for more flavor.
5. Preheat a grill or grill pan over medium-high heat.
6. Thread the marinated chicken pieces onto the soaked wooden skewers.
7. Grill the teriyaki chicken skewers for 4-5 minutes per side or until the chicken is cooked through and has grill marks.
8. While grilling, baste the chicken skewers with the reserved teriyaki marinade for added flavor.
9. Once done, transfer the grilled chicken skewers to a serving platter.
10. Garnish with sesame seeds and sliced green onions.
11. Serve the Teriyaki Chicken Skewers with rice or your preferred side dishes.

Spicy Buffalo Chicken Wraps:

Ingredients:

For Buffalo Chicken:

- 1 pound boneless, skinless chicken breasts, cooked and shredded
- 1/2 cup buffalo sauce
- 2 tablespoons unsalted butter, melted
- 1 tablespoon honey
- 1 teaspoon garlic powder
- 1/2 teaspoon onion powder

- Salt and black pepper to taste

For Wraps:

- Large flour tortillas
- Blue cheese dressing or ranch dressing
- Shredded lettuce
- Diced tomatoes
- Sliced red onion
- Avocado slices (optional)
- Fresh cilantro, chopped (for garnish)
- Lime wedges (for serving)

Instructions:

1. In a bowl, mix shredded chicken with buffalo sauce, melted butter, honey, garlic powder, onion powder, salt, and black pepper. Ensure the chicken is well coated with the buffalo sauce mixture.
2. Heat the buffalo chicken mixture in a skillet over medium heat until warmed through.
3. Place a large flour tortilla on a flat surface.
4. Spoon a portion of the buffalo chicken mixture onto the center of the tortilla.
5. Drizzle blue cheese dressing or ranch dressing over the buffalo chicken.
6. Top with shredded lettuce, diced tomatoes, sliced red onion, and avocado slices if using.
7. Garnish with chopped fresh cilantro.
8. Fold the sides of the tortilla over the filling and then roll it up tightly into a wrap.
9. Repeat the process for the remaining wraps.
10. Serve the Spicy Buffalo Chicken Wraps with lime wedges on the side.

Honey Mustard Glazed Turkey Breast:

Ingredients:

- 2 pounds turkey breast, boneless and skinless

- Salt and black pepper to taste
- 1/4 cup Dijon mustard
- 3 tablespoons honey
- 2 tablespoons whole grain mustard
- 2 tablespoons olive oil
- 2 cloves garlic, minced
- 1 teaspoon dried thyme
- 1 teaspoon paprika
- Fresh parsley, chopped (for garnish)

Instructions:

1. Preheat the oven to 375°F (190°C).
2. Season the turkey breast with salt and black pepper.
3. In a bowl, whisk together Dijon mustard, honey, whole grain mustard, olive oil, minced garlic, dried thyme, and paprika to create the honey mustard glaze.
4. Place the turkey breast in a roasting pan or on a baking sheet lined with parchment paper.
5. Brush the turkey breast with the honey mustard glaze, ensuring it is well-coated on all sides.
6. Roast in the preheated oven for about 50-60 minutes or until the internal temperature reaches 165°F (74°C) and the turkey is golden brown.
7. While roasting, baste the turkey breast with the honey mustard glaze every 20 minutes for added flavor.
8. Once done, remove the turkey breast from the oven and let it rest for 10-15 minutes before slicing.
9. Slice the turkey breast and arrange it on a serving platter.
10. Drizzle any remaining honey mustard glaze over the sliced turkey.
11. Garnish with chopped fresh parsley.
12. Serve the Honey Mustard Glazed Turkey Breast with your favorite side dishes.

Mango Habanero Grilled Chicken:

Ingredients:

- 4 boneless, skinless chicken breasts
- Salt and black pepper to taste
- 1 cup mango, peeled and diced
- 1 to 2 habanero peppers, seeds removed and minced
- 1/4 cup fresh lime juice
- 2 tablespoons honey
- 2 tablespoons soy sauce
- 2 tablespoons olive oil
- 2 cloves garlic, minced
- 1 teaspoon ground cumin
- Fresh cilantro, chopped (for garnish)
- Lime wedges (for serving)

Instructions:

1. Season the chicken breasts with salt and black pepper.
2. In a blender or food processor, combine diced mango, minced habanero peppers, fresh lime juice, honey, soy sauce, olive oil, minced garlic, and ground cumin. Blend until smooth to create the mango habanero marinade.
3. Place the chicken breasts in a shallow dish or a resealable plastic bag.
4. Pour the mango habanero marinade over the chicken, ensuring they are well-coated. Marinate in the refrigerator for at least 30 minutes, or preferably 2-4 hours for more flavor.
5. Preheat the grill to medium-high heat.
6. Remove the chicken from the refrigerator and let it come to room temperature for about 15 minutes.
7. Grill the chicken breasts for 6-8 minutes per side or until they reach an internal temperature of 165°F (74°C) and have nice grill marks.

8. While grilling, baste the chicken with any remaining mango habanero marinade for added flavor.

9. Once done, transfer the grilled chicken to a serving platter.

10. Garnish with chopped fresh cilantro.

11. Serve the Mango Habanero Grilled Chicken with lime wedges on the side.

Rosemary and Garlic Turkey Meatballs:

Ingredients:

For Turkey Meatballs:

- 1 pound ground turkey
- 1/2 cup breadcrumbs
- 1/4 cup grated Parmesan cheese
- 1/4 cup fresh parsley, chopped
- 2 cloves garlic, minced
- 1 teaspoon dried rosemary, crushed
- 1/2 teaspoon dried thyme
- 1/2 teaspoon onion powder
- 1/2 teaspoon salt
- 1/4 teaspoon black pepper
- 1 large egg, beaten
- Olive oil (for cooking)

For Sauce (Optional):

- 1 can (14 ounces) crushed tomatoes
- 2 cloves garlic, minced
- 1 teaspoon dried rosemary
- Salt and black pepper to taste

Instructions:

1. Preheat the oven to 375°F (190°C).

2. In a large bowl, combine ground turkey, breadcrumbs, grated Parmesan cheese, chopped fresh parsley, minced garlic, crushed dried rosemary, dried thyme, onion powder, salt, black pepper, and beaten egg. Mix until well combined.

3. Shape the mixture into meatballs, approximately 1 to 1.5 inches in diameter.

4. Heat olive oil in a large oven-safe skillet over medium heat.

5. Brown the meatballs on all sides in the skillet, working in batches if necessary. This step helps develop flavor and ensures the meatballs hold their shape.

6. Once browned, transfer the meatballs to the preheated oven and bake for about 15-20 minutes or until they are cooked through.

7. While the meatballs are baking, you can prepare a simple sauce. In the same skillet, add minced garlic, dried rosemary, crushed tomatoes, salt, and black pepper. Simmer for a few minutes until heated through.

8. Once the meatballs are done baking, transfer them to the skillet with the sauce if using, coating them evenly.

9. Serve the Rosemary and Garlic Turkey Meatballs on a platter, drizzling with extra sauce if desired.

Sesame Ginger Chicken Stir-Fry:

Ingredients:

For the Stir-Fry Sauce:

- 1/4 cup soy sauce
- 2 tablespoons hoisin sauce
- 1 tablespoon oyster sauce
- 1 tablespoon rice vinegar
- 1 tablespoon sesame oil
- 1 tablespoon honey
- 1 teaspoon fresh ginger, grated
- 2 cloves garlic, minced
- 1 teaspoon cornstarch (optional, for thickening)

For the Stir-Fry:

- 1 pound boneless, skinless chicken breasts, thinly sliced
- 2 tablespoons vegetable oil
- 1 bell pepper, thinly sliced
- 1 carrot, julienned
- 1 cup snap peas, trimmed
- 2 green onions, sliced
- 1 tablespoon sesame seeds (for garnish)
- Cooked rice or noodles (for serving)

Instructions:

1. In a bowl, whisk together soy sauce, hoisin sauce, oyster sauce, rice vinegar, sesame oil, honey, grated fresh ginger, minced garlic, and cornstarch (if using) to create the stir-fry sauce. Set aside.
2. Heat vegetable oil in a wok or large skillet over high heat.
3. Add sliced chicken to the hot wok and stir-fry for 3-4 minutes or until cooked through and golden brown. Remove the chicken from the wok and set aside.
4. In the same wok, add a bit more oil if needed.
5. Add sliced bell pepper, julienned carrot, and trimmed snap peas. Stir-fry for 2-3 minutes or until the vegetables are crisp-tender.
6. Return the cooked chicken to the wok.
7. Pour the stir-fry sauce over the chicken and vegetables. Toss everything together to coat evenly. If using cornstarch, the sauce will thicken as it cooks.
8. Add sliced green onions and stir-fry for an additional 1-2 minutes.
9. Sprinkle sesame seeds over the stir-fry and give it a final toss.
10. Serve the Sesame Ginger Chicken Stir-Fry over cooked rice or noodles.

Creamy Mushroom Chicken Marsala:

Ingredients:

- 4 boneless, skinless chicken breasts

- Salt and black pepper to taste
- 1/2 cup all-purpose flour, for dredging
- 4 tablespoons unsalted butter, divided
- 2 tablespoons olive oil
- 8 ounces cremini or button mushrooms, sliced
- 2 cloves garlic, minced
- 1 cup Marsala wine
- 1 cup chicken broth
- 1 cup heavy cream
- 2 tablespoons fresh parsley, chopped (for garnish)
- Cooked pasta or rice (for serving)

Instructions:

1. Season the chicken breasts with salt and black pepper.
2. Dredge each chicken breast in flour, shaking off excess.
3. In a large skillet, heat 2 tablespoons of butter and 2 tablespoons of olive oil over medium-high heat.
4. Add the chicken breasts to the skillet and cook for about 4-5 minutes per side or until they are golden brown and cooked through. Remove the chicken from the skillet and set aside.
5. In the same skillet, add the remaining 2 tablespoons of butter.
6. Add sliced mushrooms to the skillet and sauté until they release their moisture and become golden brown.
7. Stir in minced garlic and cook for an additional 1-2 minutes.
8. Pour Marsala wine into the skillet, scraping any browned bits from the bottom.
9. Add chicken broth and bring the mixture to a simmer. Cook for 5-7 minutes to allow the liquid to reduce.
10. Lower the heat and stir in heavy cream. Simmer for an additional 3-4 minutes until the sauce thickens.

11. Return the cooked chicken to the skillet, coating it with the creamy mushroom Marsala sauce.

12. Let the chicken simmer in the sauce for a couple of minutes to absorb the flavors.

13. Garnish with chopped fresh parsley.

14. Serve the Creamy Mushroom Chicken Marsala over cooked pasta or rice.

Meat Recipes:

Garlic and Herb Crusted Rack of Lamb:

Ingredients:

- 1 rack of lamb (about 1.5 to 2 pounds), frenched
- Salt and black pepper to taste
- 3 tablespoons Dijon mustard
- 3 cloves garlic, minced
- 2 tablespoons fresh rosemary, finely chopped
- 1 tablespoon fresh thyme, finely chopped
- 2 tablespoons fresh parsley, finely chopped
- 2 tablespoons olive oil
- 1 cup breadcrumbs (preferably Panko)
- 2 tablespoons unsalted butter, melted

Instructions:

1. Preheat the oven to 400°F (200°C).

2. Season the rack of lamb with salt and black pepper.

3. In a small bowl, mix Dijon mustard, minced garlic, chopped fresh rosemary, chopped fresh thyme, chopped fresh parsley, and olive oil to create the herb crust mixture.

4. Rub the herb crust mixture over the surface of the rack of lamb, ensuring it is well-coated.

5. In another bowl, combine breadcrumbs and melted butter to create the breadcrumb coating.

6. Press the breadcrumb coating onto the herb-crusted rack of lamb, covering it evenly.

7. Place the rack of lamb in a roasting pan, bone side down.

8. Roast in the preheated oven for 20-25 minutes for medium-rare, or adjust the cooking time to your desired doneness.

9. Remove the rack of lamb from the oven and let it rest for 10 minutes before slicing.

10. Slice the rack of lamb into individual chops.

11. Serve the Garlic and Herb Crusted Rack of Lamb with your favorite side dishes.

Beef and Broccoli Stir-Fry:

Ingredients:

For the Stir-Fry Sauce:

- 1/2 cup low-sodium soy sauce
- 2 tablespoons oyster sauce
- 2 tablespoons hoisin sauce
- 1 tablespoon brown sugar
- 1 tablespoon rice vinegar
- 1 tablespoon sesame oil
- 1 teaspoon cornstarch

For the Stir-Fry:

- 1 pound flank steak, thinly sliced against the grain
- 3 cups broccoli florets
- 2 tablespoons vegetable oil, divided
- 3 cloves garlic, minced
- 1 teaspoon fresh ginger, grated
- Cooked white or brown rice (for serving)

- Sesame seeds and green onions (for garnish)

Instructions:

1. In a bowl, whisk together soy sauce, oyster sauce, hoisin sauce, brown sugar, rice vinegar, sesame oil, and cornstarch to create the stir-fry sauce. Set aside.
2. Heat 1 tablespoon of vegetable oil in a wok or large skillet over medium-high heat.
3. Add sliced flank steak to the hot wok and stir-fry for 2-3 minutes or until browned and cooked to your liking. Remove the beef from the wok and set aside.
4. In the same wok, add the remaining 1 tablespoon of vegetable oil.
5. Add minced garlic and grated ginger to the wok, and stir-fry for about 30 seconds until aromatic.
6. Add broccoli florets to the wok and stir-fry for 3-4 minutes or until they are tender-crisp.
7. Return the cooked beef to the wok.
8. Pour the prepared stir-fry sauce over the beef and broccoli. Toss everything together to coat evenly.
9. Cook for an additional 1-2 minutes until the sauce thickens slightly.
10. Serve the Beef and Broccoli Stir-Fry over cooked rice.
11. Garnish with sesame seeds and sliced green onions.

Classic Beef Lasagna:

Ingredients:

For the Meat Sauce:

- 1 pound ground beef
- 1 pound Italian sausage, casings removed
- 1 onion, finely chopped
- 3 cloves garlic, minced
- 1 can (28 ounces) crushed tomatoes
- 2 cans (14 ounces each) tomato sauce
- 1 can (6 ounces) tomato paste

- 1/2 cup red wine (optional)
- 2 teaspoons dried basil
- 2 teaspoons dried oregano
- 1 teaspoon sugar
- Salt and black pepper to taste

For the Ricotta Filling:

- 2 cups ricotta cheese
- 1 cup shredded mozzarella cheese
- 1/2 cup grated Parmesan cheese
- 1 egg
- 2 tablespoons fresh parsley, chopped
- Salt and black pepper to taste

For Layering:

- 9-12 lasagna noodles, cooked according to package instructions
- 2 cups shredded mozzarella cheese
- 1/2 cup grated Parmesan cheese
- Fresh basil or parsley for garnish (optional)

Instructions:

1. Preheat the oven to 375°F (190°C).
2. In a large skillet over medium heat, brown the ground beef and Italian sausage, breaking them apart with a spoon as they cook.
3. Add finely chopped onion and minced garlic to the skillet. Cook until the onion is softened.
4. Stir in crushed tomatoes, tomato sauce, tomato paste, red wine (if using), dried basil, dried oregano, sugar, salt, and black pepper. Simmer the meat sauce for 20-30 minutes, allowing the flavors to meld.
5. In a bowl, combine ricotta cheese, shredded mozzarella cheese, grated Parmesan cheese, egg, chopped fresh parsley, salt, and black pepper. Mix well to create the ricotta filling.

6. Cook lasagna noodles according to package instructions. Drain and set aside.

7. In a large baking dish, spread a thin layer of the meat sauce.

8. Place a layer of cooked lasagna noodles over the sauce.

9. Spread half of the ricotta filling over the noodles.

10. Sprinkle it with shredded mozzarella and grated Parmesan cheese.

11. Repeat the layers: meat sauce, noodles, ricotta filling, and cheeses.

12. Finish with a final layer of noodles, meat sauce, and a generous topping of shredded mozzarella and grated Parmesan cheese.

13. Cover the baking dish with foil and bake in the preheated oven for 25-30 minutes.

14. Remove the foil and bake for an additional 10-15 minutes or until the cheese is bubbly and golden brown.

15. Let the lasagna rest for 10-15 minutes before slicing.

16. Garnish with fresh basil or parsley if desired.

Chimichurri Grilled Steak:

Ingredients:

For the Chimichurri Sauce:

- 1 cup fresh parsley, finely chopped
- 1/4 cup fresh cilantro, finely chopped
- 4 cloves garlic, minced
- 1/2 cup extra-virgin olive oil
- 3 tablespoons red wine vinegar
- 1 teaspoon dried oregano
- 1/2 teaspoon red pepper flakes (adjust to taste)
- Salt and black pepper to taste

For the Grilled Steak:

- 2 pounds sirloin, ribeye, or flank steak
- Salt and black pepper to taste
- Olive oil (for brushing)

Instructions:

1. Preheat the grill to medium-high heat.
2. Season the steak with salt and black pepper on both sides.
3. In a bowl, combine finely chopped parsley, finely chopped cilantro, minced garlic, extra-virgin olive oil, red wine vinegar, dried oregano, red pepper flakes, salt, and black pepper. Mix well to create the chimichurri sauce.
4. Set aside a portion of the chimichurri sauce for serving, and use the rest for marinating the steak.
5. Brush the steak with olive oil on both sides.
6. Generously coat the steak with the chimichurri sauce, ensuring it is well-marinated. You can let it marinate for at least 30 minutes or longer for more flavor.
7. Place the marinated steak on the preheated grill and cook to your desired doneness, usually 4-6 minutes per side for medium-rare, depending on thickness.
8. While grilling, baste the steak with additional chimichurri sauce for added flavor.
9. Once done, remove the steak from the grill and let it rest for a few minutes.
10. Slice the grilled steak against the grain.
11. Serve the Chimichurri Grilled Steak with the reserved chimichurri sauce on the side.

Moroccan Lamb Tagine:

Ingredients:

For the Spice Blend:

- 1 teaspoon ground cumin
- 1 teaspoon ground coriander
- 1 teaspoon ground cinnamon
- 1 teaspoon paprika
- 1/2 teaspoon ground ginger
- 1/2 teaspoon ground turmeric

- 1/2 teaspoon cayenne pepper (adjust to taste)
- Salt and black pepper to taste

For the Lamb Tagine:

- 2 pounds lamb shoulder, cut into chunks
- 2 tablespoons olive oil
- 1 large onion, finely chopped
- 3 cloves garlic, minced
- 1 can (14 ounces) diced tomatoes
- 1/2 cup dried apricots, chopped
- 1/2 cup raisins
- 1 tablespoon honey
- 1 cup chicken broth
- 1 preserved lemon, sliced (optional)
- Fresh cilantro, chopped (for garnish)
- Cooked couscous or rice (for serving)

Instructions:

1. In a small bowl, mix together ground cumin, ground coriander, ground cinnamon, paprika, ground ginger, ground turmeric, cayenne pepper, salt, and black pepper to create the spice blend.
2. Season the lamb chunks with the spice blend, ensuring they are well-coated. Let them marinate for at least 30 minutes.
3. In a tagine or a large, heavy-bottomed pot, heat olive oil over medium-high heat.
4. Add the marinated lamb chunks to the pot and brown on all sides.
5. Remove the browned lamb from the pot and set aside.
6. In the same pot, add chopped onion and sauté until softened.
7. Add minced garlic and sauté for an additional 1-2 minutes.
8. Return the browned lamb to the pot.
9. Stir in diced tomatoes, chopped dried apricots, raisins, honey, and chicken broth.

10. Bring the mixture to a simmer, then reduce the heat to low, cover, and let it cook for 1.5 to 2 hours or until the lamb is tender.

11. Add sliced preserved lemon to the tagine during the last 15-20 minutes of cooking, if using.

12. Adjust seasoning if needed and garnish with chopped fresh cilantro.

13. Serve the Moroccan Lamb Tagine over cooked couscous or rice.

Bacon-Wrapped Stuffed Chicken Breasts:

Ingredients:

- 4 boneless, skinless chicken breasts
- Salt and black pepper to taste
- 4 ounces cream cheese, softened
- 1/2 cup shredded cheddar cheese
- 2 green onions, finely chopped
- 1 teaspoon garlic powder
- 8 slices bacon
- Toothpicks (for securing)

Instructions:

1. Preheat the oven to 375°F (190°C).

2. Season the chicken breasts with salt and black pepper on both sides.

3. In a bowl, mix together softened cream cheese, shredded cheddar cheese, chopped green onions, and garlic powder to create the stuffing.

4. Make a horizontal cut in each chicken breast to create a pocket for the stuffing. Be careful not to cut all the way through.

5. Stuff each chicken breast with the cream cheese mixture, dividing it evenly among the breasts.

6. Wrap each stuffed chicken breast with two slices of bacon, securing the ends with toothpicks.

7. Heat a skillet over medium-high heat. Sear the bacon-wrapped chicken breasts on all sides until the bacon is browned.

8. Transfer the seared chicken breasts to a baking dish.

9. Bake in the preheated oven for 25-30 minutes or until the chicken is cooked through and reaches an internal temperature of 165°F (74°C).

10. If desired, broil the chicken for an additional 2-3 minutes to crisp up the bacon.

11. Carefully remove toothpicks before serving.

Pork Tenderloin with Apple Chutney:

Ingredients:

For the Pork Tenderloin:

- 2 pork tenderloins (about 1 to 1.5 pounds each)
- Salt and black pepper to taste
- 2 tablespoons olive oil
- 2 teaspoons dried thyme or rosemary (optional)

For the Apple Chutney:

- 2 apples, peeled, cored, and diced
- 1/2 cup red onion, finely chopped
- 1/4 cup dried cranberries or raisins
- 1/4 cup brown sugar
- 1/4 cup apple cider vinegar
- 1 teaspoon ground cinnamon
- 1/2 teaspoon ground ginger
- 1/4 teaspoon ground cloves
- Salt and black pepper to taste

Instructions:

1. Preheat the oven to 375°F (190°C).

2. Season the pork tenderloins with salt, black pepper, and dried thyme or rosemary if using.

3. In an oven-safe skillet, heat olive oil over medium-high heat.

4. Sear the pork tenderloins on all sides until browned.

5. Transfer the skillet to the preheated oven and roast for about 20-25 minutes or until the internal temperature reaches 145°F (63°C) for medium doneness.

6. While the pork is roasting, prepare the apple chutney.

7. In a saucepan over medium heat, combine diced apples, chopped red onion, dried cranberries or raisins, brown sugar, apple cider vinegar, ground cinnamon, ground ginger, ground cloves, salt, and black pepper.

8. Cook the apple chutney for about 10-15 minutes or until the apples are tender and the mixture has thickened.

9. Adjust the seasoning of the chutney to taste.

10. Once the pork tenderloins are done, remove them from the oven and let them rest for a few minutes.

11. Slice the pork tenderloins into medallions and serve with the apple chutney.

12. Garnish with additional fresh herbs if desired.

13. Serve the Pork Tenderloin with Apple Chutney with your favorite side dishes.

Italian Sausage and Peppers:

Ingredients:

- 1 pound Italian sausage links (sweet or hot)
- 2 tablespoons olive oil
- 1 large onion, thinly sliced
- 2 bell peppers, thinly sliced (assorted colors)
- 3 cloves garlic, minced
- 1 can (14 ounces) crushed tomatoes
- 1 teaspoon dried oregano
- 1 teaspoon dried basil
- Salt and black pepper to taste
- Red pepper flakes (optional, for added heat)

- Fresh parsley, chopped (for garnish)
- Crusty Italian bread or rolls (for serving)

Instructions:

1. In a large skillet or pan, heat olive oil over medium heat.
2. Add the Italian sausage links to the skillet and brown them on all sides. Cook until they are cooked through, about 10-12 minutes.
3. Once the sausages are cooked, remove them from the skillet and set aside.
4. In the same skillet, add sliced onions and bell peppers. Sauté until they are softened and slightly caramelized.
5. Add minced garlic to the skillet and cook for an additional 1-2 minutes until fragrant.
6. Pour in crushed tomatoes, dried oregano, dried basil, salt, black pepper, and red pepper flakes if using. Stir to combine.
7. Cut the cooked Italian sausages into slices and add them back to the skillet.
8. Simmer the sausage and pepper mixture for 10-15 minutes, allowing the flavors to meld.
9. Adjust seasoning to taste.
10. Garnish with chopped fresh parsley.
11. Serve the Italian Sausage and Peppers over pasta, rice, or with crusty Italian bread or rolls.

Spaghetti Bolognese:

Ingredients:

- 1 pound ground beef
- 1 tablespoon olive oil
- 1 onion, finely chopped
- 2 carrots, peeled and finely chopped
- 2 celery stalks, finely chopped
- 3 cloves garlic, minced

- 1/2 cup red wine (optional)
- 1 can (28 ounces) crushed tomatoes
- 2 tablespoons tomato paste
- 1 teaspoon dried oregano
- 1 teaspoon dried basil
- 1/2 teaspoon dried thyme
- 1 bay leaf
- Salt and black pepper to taste
- 1/2 cup whole milk or heavy cream
- 1 pound spaghetti
- Grated Parmesan cheese (for serving)
- Fresh basil or parsley, chopped (for garnish)

Instructions:

1. Heat olive oil in a large pot or Dutch oven over medium heat.
2. Add the ground beef and cook until browned, breaking it apart with a spoon as it cooks.
3. Add finely chopped onion, carrots, and celery to the pot. Sauté until the vegetables are softened.
4. Stir in minced garlic and cook for an additional 1-2 minutes until fragrant.
5. If using, pour in red wine to deglaze the pot, scraping up any browned bits from the bottom.
6. Add crushed tomatoes, tomato paste, dried oregano, dried basil, dried thyme, bay leaf, salt, and black pepper. Mix well.
7. Bring the mixture to a simmer, then reduce the heat to low and let it cook for 1 to 1.5 hours, stirring occasionally to allow the flavors to meld.
8. Pour in the whole milk or heavy cream and stir to combine. Simmer for an additional 15-20 minutes.
9. Meanwhile, cook the spaghetti according to package instructions. Drain and set aside.

10. Taste and adjust the seasoning of the Bolognese sauce as needed.

11. Discard the bay leaf.

12. Serve the Bolognese sauce over the cooked spaghetti.

Barbecue Pulled Pork Sandwiches:

Ingredients:

For the Pulled Pork:

- 3-4 pounds pork shoulder or pork butt
- 2 tablespoons brown sugar
- 1 tablespoon paprika
- 1 tablespoon garlic powder
- 1 tablespoon onion powder
- 1 teaspoon cayenne pepper
- 1 teaspoon ground cumin
- Salt and black pepper to taste
- 1 cup barbecue sauce (plus extra for serving)
- 1 cup chicken or vegetable broth

For the Coleslaw (Optional, for topping):

- 2 cups shredded cabbage
- 1 carrot, grated
- 1/2 cup mayonnaise
- 1 tablespoon apple cider vinegar
- 1 tablespoon honey
- Salt and black pepper to taste

For Serving:

- Hamburger buns or sandwich rolls

Instructions:

1. Preheat the oven to 300°F (150°C).

2. In a small bowl, mix brown sugar, paprika, garlic powder, onion powder, cayenne pepper, ground cumin, salt, and black pepper to create a dry rub.

3. Rub the dry rub all over the pork shoulder or pork butt, ensuring it is well-coated.

4. Place the seasoned pork in a roasting pan or Dutch oven.

5. Mix barbecue sauce and broth together, then pour the mixture over the pork.

6. Cover the roasting pan or Dutch oven with a lid or tightly with foil.

7. Roast in the preheated oven for 4-6 hours or until the pork is fork-tender and easily pulls apart.

8. Once cooked, shred the pork using two forks, discarding any excess fat.

9. If making coleslaw, mix shredded cabbage, grated carrot, mayonnaise, apple cider vinegar, honey, salt, and black pepper in a bowl. Refrigerate until ready to use.

10. Toast the hamburger buns or sandwich rolls.

11. Assemble the barbecue pulled pork sandwiches by placing a generous amount of pulled pork on the bottom half of each bun.

12. Top with additional barbecue sauce and coleslaw if desired.

13. Cover with the top half of the bun.

14. Serve the Barbecue Pulled Pork Sandwiches immediately.

Maple Dijon Glazed Ham:

Ingredients:

- 1 fully-cooked ham (bone-in or boneless, about 6-8 pounds)
- 1/2 cup maple syrup
- 1/4 cup Dijon mustard
- 1/4 cup brown sugar
- 2 tablespoons apple cider vinegar
- 1 teaspoon ground cinnamon
- 1/2 teaspoon ground cloves
- 1/4 teaspoon black pepper

Instructions:

1. Preheat the oven to 325°F (163°C).

2. Place the ham in a roasting pan, and score the surface with shallow cuts in a diamond pattern.

3. In a bowl, whisk together maple syrup, Dijon mustard, brown sugar, apple cider vinegar, ground cinnamon, ground cloves, and black pepper to create the glaze.

4. Brush the glaze generously over the surface of the ham, making sure to get into the scored cuts.

5. Tent the ham with foil and bake in the preheated oven for about 15-20 minutes per pound, or according to the package instructions for your specific ham.

6. Every 30 minutes, baste the ham with the drippings and glaze.

7. About 30 minutes before the ham is done, remove the foil to allow the glaze to caramelize and create a golden brown finish.

8. Once the ham reaches an internal temperature of 140°F (60°C), remove it from the oven.

9. Let the Maple Dijon Glazed Ham rest for about 15 minutes before carving.

10. Slice and serve the ham, drizzling any remaining glaze over the slices.

11. Optionally, serve with additional glaze on the side.

Berry Blast Smoothie:

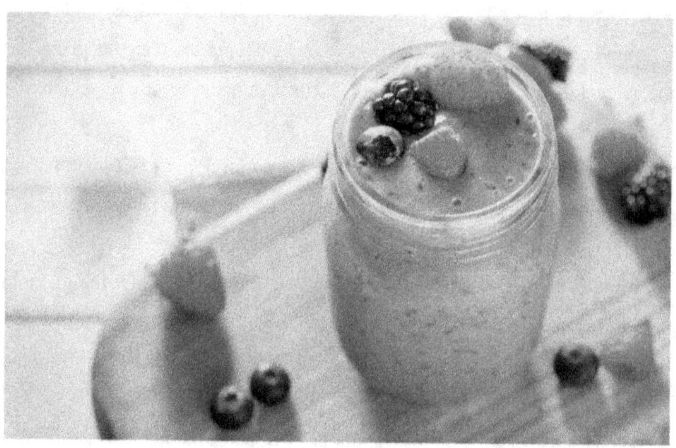

Ingredients:

- 1 cup mixed berries (such as blueberries, strawberries, and raspberries)
- 1/2 banana
- 1/2 cup plain Greek yogurt
- 1/2 cup almond milk (or any non-dairy milk)
- 1 tablespoon chia seeds
- 1 tablespoon flaxseeds
- 1 teaspoon honey (optional, for sweetness)
- Ice cubes (optional)

Instructions:

1. Wash the berries thoroughly.
2. In a blender, combine the mixed berries, banana, Greek yogurt, almond milk, chia seeds, flaxseeds, and honey.
3. Blend on high until smooth and creamy.

4. If the smoothie is too thick, add more almond milk until you reach your desired consistency.

5. Taste and adjust sweetness by adding more honey if needed.

6. If you prefer a colder smoothie, add ice cubes and blend again until smooth.

7. Pour the Berry Blast Smoothie into a glass and enjoy!

Green Mango Tango:

Ingredients:

- 1 ripe green mango, peeled and diced
- 1 cup spinach leaves
- 1/2 cucumber, peeled and sliced
- 1/2 green apple, cored and chopped
- 1/2 lime, juiced
- 1 tablespoon fresh mint leaves
- 1 cup coconut water
- Ice cubes (optional)

Instructions:

1. In a blender, combine the diced green mango, spinach leaves, sliced cucumber, chopped green apple, lime juice, and fresh mint leaves.

2. Pour in the coconut water to the blender.

3. Blend the ingredients on high until smooth and well combined.

4. If the smoothie is too thick, add more coconut water until you achieve your desired consistency.

5. Taste the Green Mango Tango and adjust the flavor by adding more lime juice if needed.

6. For a colder version, add ice cubes and blend again until smooth.

7. Pour the Green Mango Tango into a glass and garnish with additional mint leaves if desired.

Pineapple Paradise Smoothie:

Ingredients:

- 1 cup fresh pineapple chunks
- 1/2 banana
- 1/2 cup coconut milk
- 1/2 cup orange juice
- 1/2 cup Greek yogurt
- 1 tablespoon chia seeds
- Ice cubes (optional)

Instructions:

1. Cut fresh pineapple into chunks.
2. In a blender, combine the pineapple chunks, banana, coconut milk, orange juice, Greek yogurt, and chia seeds.
3. Blend on high speed until the mixture is smooth and creamy.
4. If the smoothie is too thick, add more coconut milk or orange juice to reach your preferred consistency.
5. Taste the Pineapple Paradise Smoothie and adjust sweetness by adding more banana if needed.
6. Optionally, add ice cubes and blend again for a colder and thicker texture.
7. Pour the smoothie into a glass and enjoy the tropical goodness.

Choco-Berry Protein Smoothie:

Ingredients:

- 1 cup mixed berries (such as strawberries, blueberries, and raspberries)
- 1 banana
- 1 cup unsweetened almond milk
- 1 scoop chocolate protein powder
- 1 tablespoon almond butter
- 1 tablespoon chia seeds

- Ice cubes (optional)

Instructions:

1. Wash the mixed berries thoroughly.
2. In a blender, combine the mixed berries, banana, almond milk, chocolate protein powder, almond butter, and chia seeds.
3. Blend on high speed until the ingredients are well combined and the smoothie is creamy.
4. If the smoothie is too thick, add more almond milk until you reach the desired consistency.
5. Taste and adjust sweetness by adding more banana or a touch of honey if needed.
6. Optionally, add ice cubes and blend again for a colder and thicker texture.
7. Pour the Choco-Berry Protein Smoothie into a glass and enjoy this delicious and protein-packed treat.

Tropical Turmeric Smoothie:

Ingredients:

- 1 cup pineapple chunks
- 1/2 mango, peeled and diced
- 1/2 banana
- 1/2 teaspoon ground turmeric
- 1/2 teaspoon grated fresh ginger
- 1 cup coconut water
- 1 tablespoon chia seeds
- Ice cubes (optional)

Instructions:

1. Cut fresh pineapple into chunks and peel and dice the mango.
2. In a blender, combine the pineapple chunks, diced mango, banana, ground turmeric, grated fresh ginger, coconut water, and chia seeds.
3. Blend on high speed until the mixture is smooth and well combined.

4. If the smoothie is too thick, add more coconut water until you achieve the desired consistency.

5. Taste the Tropical Turmeric Smoothie and adjust the flavor by adding more ginger or a splash of lime juice if desired.

6. Optionally, add ice cubes and blend again for a colder and refreshing texture.

7. Pour the smoothie into a glass and savor the tropical and anti-inflammatory goodness.

Peachy Green Tea Smoothie:

Ingredients:

- 1 ripe peach, pitted and sliced
- 1/2 banana
- 1 cup baby spinach leaves
- 1 cup brewed green tea, cooled
- 1/2 cup plain Greek yogurt
- 1 tablespoon honey
- Ice cubes (optional)

Instructions:

1. Pit and slice the ripe peach.

2. In a blender, combine the peach slices, banana, baby spinach leaves, brewed green tea, Greek yogurt, and honey.

3. Blend on high speed until the ingredients are well combined and the smoothie is creamy.

4. If the smoothie is too thick, add more brewed green tea until you reach the desired consistency.

5. Taste and adjust sweetness by adding more honey if needed.

6. Optionally, add ice cubes and blend again for a colder and more refreshing texture.

7. Pour the Peachy Green Tea Smoothie into a glass and enjoy the delightful combination of peach, green tea, and spinach.

Creamy Avocado Lime Smoothie:

Ingredients:

- 1 ripe avocado, peeled and pitted
- 1 banana
- 1 cup spinach leaves
- 1/2 cup plain Greek yogurt
- Juice of 2 limes
- 1-2 tablespoons honey (optional, for sweetness)
- 1 cup almond milk (or any non-dairy milk)
- Ice cubes (optional)

Instructions:

1. In a blender, combine the peeled and pitted avocado, banana, spinach leaves, Greek yogurt, lime juice, and honey.
2. Add almond milk to the blender.
3. Blend on high speed until the mixture is smooth and creamy.
4. If the smoothie is too thick, add more almond milk until you reach your preferred consistency.
5. Taste the Creamy Avocado Lime Smoothie and adjust sweetness by adding more honey if needed.
6. Optionally, add ice cubes and blend again for a colder and thicker texture.
7. Pour the smoothie into a glass and savor the creamy and refreshing goodness.

Strawberry Banana Oat Smoothie:

Ingredients:

- 1 cup strawberries, hulled and halved
- 1 banana
- 1/2 cup rolled oats
- 1/2 cup plain Greek yogurt
- 1 cup milk (dairy or plant-based)

- 1 tablespoon honey or maple syrup (optional, for sweetness)
- Ice cubes (optional)

Instructions:

1. Hull and halve the strawberries.
2. In a blender, combine the strawberries, banana, rolled oats, Greek yogurt, milk, and honey (if using).
3. Blend on high speed until the ingredients are well combined and the smoothie is creamy.
4. If the smoothie is too thick, add more milk until you reach your desired consistency.
5. Taste and adjust sweetness by adding more honey if needed.
6. Optionally, add ice cubes and blend again for a colder and thicker texture.
7. Pour the Strawberry Banana Oat Smoothie into a glass and enjoy this wholesome and satisfying drink.

Minty Watermelon Refresher:

Ingredients:

- 2 cups diced seedless watermelon
- 1/2 cucumber, peeled and sliced
- 1/4 cup fresh mint leaves
- Juice of 1 lime
- 1-2 tablespoons honey or agave syrup (optional, for sweetness)
- 1 cup cold water
- Ice cubes (optional)

Instructions:

1. Dice seedless watermelon and peel and slice the cucumber.
2. In a blender, combine the diced watermelon, sliced cucumber, fresh mint leaves, lime juice, and honey (if using).
3. Add cold water to the blender.

4. Blend on high speed until the mixture is smooth and well combined.

5. If the refresher is too thick, add more water until you reach your desired consistency.

6. Taste and adjust sweetness by adding more honey if needed.

7. Optionally, add ice cubes and blend again for a colder and more refreshing texture.

8. Pour the Minty Watermelon Refresher into a glass, garnish with mint leaves, and enjoy this hydrating and mint-infused treat.

Coffee and Almond Butter Energizer:

Ingredients:

- 1 cup brewed coffee, cooled
- 1 banana
- 2 tablespoons almond butter
- 1 tablespoon honey or maple syrup (optional, for sweetness)
- 1/2 cup milk (dairy or plant-based)
- Ice cubes (optional)

Instructions:

1. Brew a cup of coffee and let it cool to room temperature.

2. In a blender, combine the cooled brewed coffee, banana, almond butter, honey (if using), and milk.

3. Blend on high speed until the ingredients are well combined and the smoothie is creamy.

4. If the smoothie is too thick, add more milk until you reach your desired consistency.

5. Taste and adjust sweetness by adding more honey if needed.

6. Optionally, add ice cubes and blend again for a colder and more invigorating texture.

7. Pour the Coffee and Almond Butter Energizer into a glass and kickstart your day with this energizing coffee-infused smoothie.

Dark Chocolate Avocado Mousse:

Ingredients:

- **2 ripe avocados**, peeled and pitted
- 1/4 cup unsweetened cocoa powder
- 1/4 cup dark chocolate chips, melted
- 1/4 cup maple syrup or agave nectar
- 1 teaspoon vanilla extract
- Pinch of salt
- Fresh berries or mint leaves for garnish (optional)

Instructions:

1. In a food processor, combine the peeled and pitted avocados, cocoa powder, melted dark chocolate chips, maple syrup (or agave nectar), vanilla extract, and a pinch of salt.
2. Blend the ingredients until smooth and creamy, scraping down the sides of the processor as needed.
3. Taste the mousse and adjust sweetness by adding more maple syrup if desired.
4. Once the mixture is well combined, transfer the Dark Chocolate Avocado Mousse into serving bowls or glasses.
5. Refrigerate the mousse for at least 1-2 hours to allow it to set.
6. Before serving, garnish with fresh berries or mint leaves if desired.
7. Enjoy this rich and indulgent Dark Chocolate Avocado Mousse as a guilt-free dessert or treat.

Coconut Chia Pudding:

Ingredients:

- 1/4 cup chia seeds
- 1 cup coconut milk

- 1 tablespoon maple syrup or agave nectar
- 1/2 teaspoon vanilla extract
- Shredded coconut and fresh berries for topping (optional)

Instructions:

1. In a bowl, combine the chia seeds, coconut milk, maple syrup (or agave nectar), and vanilla extract.
2. Whisk the ingredients together thoroughly to ensure the chia seeds are well distributed.
3. Cover the bowl and refrigerate for at least 3-4 hours or overnight to allow the chia seeds to absorb the liquid and create a pudding-like consistency.
4. Stir the Coconut Chia Pudding well before serving to break up any clumps.
5. If the pudding is too thick, you can add a little more coconut milk to reach your desired consistency.
6. Spoon the chia pudding into serving glasses or bowls.
7. Optionally, top with shredded coconut and fresh berries for added texture and flavor.
8. Enjoy this simple and delicious Coconut Chia Pudding as a nutritious breakfast or satisfying dessert.

Baked Apple with Cinnamon:

Ingredients:

- 2 apples (such as Granny Smith or Honeycrisp)
- 1 tablespoon melted butter or coconut oil
- 1 tablespoon honey or maple syrup
- 1 teaspoon ground cinnamon
- 1/4 cup chopped nuts (such as walnuts or pecans, optional)
- Vanilla ice cream or yogurt for serving (optional)

Instructions:

1. Preheat the oven to 375°F (190°C).

2. Wash and core the apples, leaving the bottoms intact.

3. Place the apples in a baking dish.

4. In a small bowl, mix the melted butter or coconut oil, honey (or maple syrup), and ground cinnamon until well combined.

5. Brush the mixture over the apples, ensuring they are well coated.

6. If desired, sprinkle chopped nuts over the top of each apple.

7. Bake in the preheated oven for 25-30 minutes or until the apples are tender and have a golden-brown color.

8. Remove from the oven and let them cool slightly before serving.

9. Optionally, serve the Baked Apples with a scoop of vanilla ice cream or a dollop of yogurt for a delightful treat.

Vegan Chocolate Banana Ice Cream:

Ingredients:

- 4 ripe bananas, peeled, sliced, and frozen
- 3 tablespoons unsweetened cocoa powder
- 2 tablespoons maple syrup or agave nectar
- 1 teaspoon vanilla extract
- A pinch of salt
- Plant-based milk (such as almond or coconut) as needed

Instructions:

1. Slice ripe bananas and freeze them until solid (at least 4 hours or overnight).

2. In a food processor or high-powered blender, add the frozen banana slices, cocoa powder, maple syrup (or agave nectar), vanilla extract, and a pinch of salt.

3. Start blending on low speed, gradually increasing to high. Use a spatula to scrape down the sides if needed.

4. If the mixture is too thick and difficult to blend, add a splash of plant-based milk to help achieve a smoother consistency.

5. Continue blending until the Vegan Chocolate Banana Ice Cream is smooth and creamy.

6. Taste the ice cream and adjust sweetness if necessary by adding more maple syrup.

7. Transfer the ice cream to a container and freeze for an additional 1-2 hours if a firmer texture is preferred.

8. Scoop and serve this dairy-free delight, enjoying the rich and creamy goodness guilt-free.

Lemon Blueberry Parfait:

Ingredients:

- 1 cup fresh blueberries
- 2 tablespoons lemon juice
- 2 tablespoons honey or maple syrup
- 1 cup Greek yogurt (or coconut yogurt for a vegan option)
- 1 teaspoon lemon zest
- 1 cup granola

Instructions:

1. In a small saucepan, combine the fresh blueberries, lemon juice, and honey (or maple syrup).

2. Cook over medium heat for 5-7 minutes, stirring occasionally, until the blueberries soften and release their juices. Allow the mixture to cool.

3. In a bowl, mix the Greek yogurt with lemon zest until well combined.

4. In serving glasses or bowls, layer the Lemon Blueberry Parfait. Start with a spoonful of the yogurt mixture, followed by a layer of the blueberry compote, and then a layer of granola.

5. Repeat the layers until the glasses are filled, finishing with a dollop of the yogurt mixture on top.

6. Optionally, garnish with additional blueberries and a sprinkle of granola.

7. Refrigerate for at least 30 minutes before serving to allow the flavors to meld.

8. Enjoy this refreshing and delightful Lemon Blueberry Parfait

Almond Joy Energy Bites:

Ingredients:

- 1 cup rolled oats
- 1/2 cup almond butter
- 1/4 cup honey or maple syrup
- 1/4 cup shredded coconut (plus extra for rolling)
- 1/4 cup chopped almonds
- 2 tablespoons cocoa powder
- 1 teaspoon vanilla extract
- A pinch of salt

Instructions:

1. In a large mixing bowl, combine rolled oats, almond butter, honey (or maple syrup), shredded coconut, chopped almonds, cocoa powder, vanilla extract, and a pinch of salt.
2. Mix the ingredients thoroughly until well combined.
3. Place the bowl in the refrigerator for 15-30 minutes to allow the mixture to firm up, making it easier to shape into bites.
4. Once chilled, take small portions of the mixture and roll them into bite-sized balls.
5. Roll each energy bite in additional shredded coconut to coat the surface.
6. Place the Almond Joy Energy Bites on a parchment-lined tray or plate.
7. Refrigerate for at least 30 minutes before serving to allow the bites to set.
8. Store the energy bites in an airtight container in the refrigerator.

Raspberry Coconut Popsicles:

Ingredients:

- 1 cup fresh raspberries
- 1/2 cup coconut milk

- 1/2 cup Greek yogurt (or coconut yogurt for a dairy-free option)
- 2 tablespoons honey or maple syrup
- 1 teaspoon vanilla extract
- Shredded coconut (optional, for coating)

Instructions:

1. In a blender, combine fresh raspberries, coconut milk, Greek yogurt (or coconut yogurt), honey (or maple syrup), and vanilla extract.
2. Blend the mixture until smooth and well combined.
3. Taste the raspberry coconut mixture and adjust sweetness if needed by adding more honey or maple syrup.
4. Pour the mixture into popsicle molds, leaving a little space at the top for expansion.
5. If desired, sprinkle shredded coconut on top of each popsicle or roll the popsicles in shredded coconut.
6. Insert popsicle sticks into each mold and freeze for at least 4-6 hours, or until the popsicles are completely frozen.
7. Once frozen, run the molds under warm water for a few seconds to release the Raspberry Coconut Popsicles.
8. Enjoy these refreshing and naturally sweet popsicles on a hot day!

Strawberry Shortcake Cups:

Ingredients:

- 2 cups fresh strawberries, hulled and sliced
- 2 tablespoons sugar
- 1 cup heavy cream
- 2 tablespoons powdered sugar
- 1 teaspoon vanilla extract
- Shortcake cups or angel food cake, sliced into cubes

Instructions:

1. In a bowl, combine sliced strawberries and sugar. Toss gently to coat the strawberries and let them sit for about 15 minutes to macerate.

2. In a separate bowl, whip the heavy cream until it starts to thicken.

3. Add powdered sugar and vanilla extract to the whipped cream. Continue whipping until stiff peaks form.

4. Gently fold the macerated strawberries into the whipped cream, reserving a few for garnish.

5. In serving cups or bowls, layer shortcake cubes followed by the strawberry and cream mixture.

6. Repeat the layers, finishing with a dollop of the strawberry and cream mixture on top.

7. Garnish with reserved strawberries.

8. Refrigerate for at least 30 minutes before serving to allow the flavors to meld.

9. Serve chilled and enjoy these delightful Strawberry Shortcake Cups.

Pumpkin Spice Chia Seed Pudding:

Ingredients:

- 1/4 cup chia seeds
- 1 cup unsweetened almond milk (or any milk of your choice)
- 1/2 cup pumpkin puree
- 2 tablespoons maple syrup or honey
- 1/2 teaspoon pumpkin spice blend (cinnamon, nutmeg, ginger, and cloves)
- 1/2 teaspoon vanilla extract
- Optional toppings: chopped nuts, pumpkin seeds, or a dollop of whipped cream

Instructions:

1. In a bowl, whisk together chia seeds and almond milk.

2. Add pumpkin puree, maple syrup (or honey), pumpkin spice blend, and vanilla extract to the chia seed mixture.

3. Whisk everything together until well combined.

4. Cover the bowl and refrigerate for at least 3-4 hours or overnight to allow the chia seeds to absorb the liquid and create a pudding-like consistency.

5. Stir the Pumpkin Spice Chia Seed Pudding well before serving to ensure an even texture.

6. If the pudding is too thick, you can add a little more almond milk to reach your desired consistency.

7. Spoon the pudding into serving glasses or bowls.

8. Optionally, top with chopped nuts, pumpkin seeds, or a dollop of whipped cream for added texture and flavor.

9. Enjoy this festive and nutritious Pumpkin Spice Chia Seed Pudding as a flavorful dessert or breakfast treat.

Banana Nut Oat Cookies:

Ingredients:

- 2 ripe bananas, mashed
- 1 cup rolled oats
- 1/2 cup chopped nuts (walnuts, pecans, or almonds)
- 1/4 cup almond butter or peanut butter
- 1/4 cup honey or maple syrup
- 1 teaspoon vanilla extract
- 1/2 teaspoon ground cinnamon
- 1/4 teaspoon salt

Instructions:

1. Preheat the oven to 350°F (175°C). Line a baking sheet with parchment paper.

2. In a large bowl, combine mashed bananas, rolled oats, chopped nuts, almond butter (or peanut butter), honey (or maple syrup), vanilla extract, ground cinnamon, and salt.

3. Mix the ingredients until well combined and a dough forms.

4. Drop spoonfuls of the cookie dough onto the prepared baking sheet, spacing them apart.

5. Use the back of a fork to flatten each cookie slightly.

6. Bake in the preheated oven for 12-15 minutes or until the edges are golden brown.

7. Remove from the oven and allow the Banana Nut Oat Cookies to cool on the baking sheet for a few minutes before transferring them to a wire rack to cool completely.

8. Once cooled, store the cookies in an airtight container.

Mixed Berry Sorbet:

Ingredients:

- 3 cups mixed berries (strawberries, blueberries, raspberries)
- 1/2 cup granulated sugar
- 1 tablespoon fresh lemon juice
- 1/2 cup water

Instructions:

1. Wash the mixed berries thoroughly and remove any stems.

2. In a small saucepan, combine sugar and water over medium heat. Stir until the sugar is completely dissolved, creating a simple syrup. Allow it to cool.

3. In a blender or food processor, combine the mixed berries and fresh lemon juice.

4. Blend until the berries are pureed.

5. Add the cooled simple syrup to the berry puree and blend again until well combined.

6. Strain the mixture through a fine-mesh sieve to remove seeds and pulp, if desired.

7. Pour the sorbet mixture into an ice cream maker and churn according to the manufacturer's instructions.

8. Once churned, transfer the sorbet to a lidded container and freeze for at least 4 hours or until firm.

9. Before serving, allow the Mixed Berry Sorbet to soften slightly at room
   temperature for easier scooping.

CHAPTER 9: CONDIMENTS, DRESSINGS AND SAUCES

Homemade Ketchup:

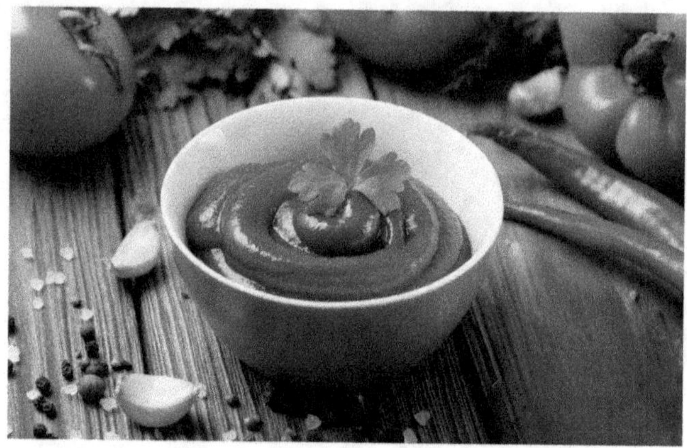

Ingredients:

- 1 can (28 ounces) crushed tomatoes
- 1/2 cup white vinegar
- 1/4 cup brown sugar
- 1 teaspoon onion powder
- 1 teaspoon garlic powder
- 1 teaspoon salt
- 1/2 teaspoon mustard powder
- 1/4 teaspoon ground cloves
- 1/4 teaspoon allspice

Instructions:

1. In a medium saucepan, combine the crushed tomatoes, white vinegar, brown sugar, onion powder, garlic powder, salt, mustard powder, ground cloves, and allspice.
2. Bring the mixture to a simmer over medium heat.

3. Reduce the heat to low and let it simmer for about 1 to 1.5 hours, stirring occasionally, until the ketchup thickens.

4. Taste the ketchup and adjust the seasoning if needed. You can add more sugar for sweetness or more salt for seasoning.

5. Once the ketchup reaches your desired thickness, remove it from the heat and let it cool to room temperature.

6. Use an immersion blender or transfer the mixture to a regular blender to blend until smooth.

7. Pour the Homemade Ketchup into a sterilized jar or bottle.

8. Refrigerate for at least a few hours before using to allow the flavors to meld.

Spicy Mango Salsa:

Ingredients:

- 2 ripe mangoes, peeled, pitted, and diced
- 1/2 red onion, finely chopped
- 1 red bell pepper, diced
- 1 jalapeño pepper, finely chopped (seeds removed for milder heat)
- 1/4 cup fresh cilantro, chopped
- Juice of 2 limes
- Salt to taste

Instructions:

1. In a bowl, combine the diced mangoes, chopped red onion, diced red bell pepper, chopped jalapeño pepper, and chopped cilantro.

2. Squeeze the juice of two limes over the ingredients.

3. Mix the ingredients thoroughly until well combined.

4. Taste the Spicy Mango Salsa and add salt as needed.

5. Cover the bowl and refrigerate for at least 30 minutes to allow the flavors to meld.

6. Before serving, give the salsa a final stir and adjust lime or salt if necessary.

7. Serve the Spicy Mango Salsa with tortilla chips, grilled chicken, fish, or as a topping for tacos.

Garlic Aioli:

Ingredients:

- 1 cup mayonnaise
- 3 cloves garlic, minced
- 1 tablespoon lemon juice
- 1/2 teaspoon Dijon mustard
- Salt and pepper to taste

Instructions:

1. In a bowl, combine mayonnaise, minced garlic, lemon juice, and Dijon mustard.
2. Mix the ingredients thoroughly until the garlic is evenly distributed.
3. Season the Garlic Aioli with salt and pepper to taste.
4. Taste and adjust the flavor by adding more garlic, lemon juice, mustard, salt, or pepper according to your preference.
5. Cover the bowl and refrigerate the aioli for at least 30 minutes before serving to allow the flavors to meld.
6. Serve the Garlic Aioli as a dipping sauce for fries, vegetables, or seafood, or as a flavorful spread for sandwiches and burgers.

Chipotle Mayo:

Ingredients:

- 1 cup mayonnaise
- 1-2 tablespoons adobo sauce from a can of chipotle peppers in adobo
- 1 tablespoon lime juice
- 1 teaspoon honey
- Salt to taste

Instructions:

1. In a bowl, combine mayonnaise, adobo sauce, lime juice, and honey.

2. Mix the ingredients thoroughly until the adobo sauce is evenly distributed.

3. Taste the Chipotle Mayo and add salt if needed.

4. Adjust the flavor by adding more adobo sauce for extra heat or honey for sweetness, according to your preference.

5. Cover the bowl and refrigerate the chipotle mayo for at least 30 minutes before serving to allow the flavors to meld.

6. Serve the Chipotle Mayo as a spicy and smoky dipping sauce, or use it as a zesty spread for sandwiches, burgers, or wraps.

Pickled Red Onions:

Ingredients:

- 1 large red onion, thinly sliced
- 1 cup apple cider vinegar
- 1 cup water
- 2 tablespoons sugar
- 1 tablespoon salt
- Optional: 1 teaspoon whole black peppercorns, 1-2 cloves, or a pinch of red pepper flakes for added flavor

Instructions:

1. Peel and thinly slice the red onion into rings or half-moons.

2. In a saucepan, combine apple cider vinegar, water, sugar, salt, and any optional spices you choose.

3. Bring the mixture to a simmer over medium heat, stirring to dissolve the sugar and salt.

4. Place the sliced red onions in a clean glass jar or container.

5. Pour the hot vinegar mixture over the onions, ensuring they are fully submerged.

6. Let the Pickled Red Onions cool to room temperature.

7. Once cooled, cover the jar or container and refrigerate for at least 1-2 hours before using to allow the flavors to develop.

8. The pickled onions can be stored in the refrigerator for up to a few weeks.

Cilantro Lime Crema:

Ingredients:

- 1 cup sour cream
- 1/4 cup fresh cilantro, finely chopped
- 1 tablespoon lime juice
- 1 teaspoon lime zest
- 1 clove garlic, minced
- Salt and pepper to taste

Instructions:

1. In a bowl, combine sour cream, chopped cilantro, lime juice, lime zest, and minced garlic.

2. Mix the ingredients thoroughly until the cilantro and garlic are evenly distributed.

3. Season the Cilantro Lime Crema with salt and pepper to taste.

4. Taste and adjust the flavor by adding more lime juice, cilantro, garlic, salt, or pepper according to your preference.

5. Cover the bowl and refrigerate the crema for at least 30 minutes before serving to allow the flavors to meld.

6. Serve the Cilantro Lime Crema as a refreshing and zesty topping for tacos, quesadillas, grilled meats, or as a dipping sauce for veggies.

Homemade Mustard:

Ingredients:

- 1/2 cup yellow mustard seeds
- 1/2 cup brown mustard seeds
- 1 cup white wine vinegar

- 1/2 cup water
- 1 teaspoon salt
- 1/2 teaspoon turmeric powder
- 1/4 teaspoon garlic powder
- Optional: honey or maple syrup for sweetness, to taste

Instructions:

1. In a bowl, combine yellow and brown mustard seeds with white wine vinegar and water.
2. Cover the bowl and let the mustard seeds soak at room temperature for at least 24 hours to soften.
3. After soaking, transfer the soaked mustard seeds to a blender or food processor.
4. Add salt, turmeric powder, and garlic powder to the blender.
5. Blend the mixture until you reach your desired mustard consistency. You can adjust the texture by adding more water if needed.
6. Taste the Homemade Mustard and adjust the flavor by adding honey or maple syrup for sweetness, if desired.
7. Transfer the mustard to a sterilized jar and refrigerate for at least 24 hours before using to allow the flavors to meld.

Sriracha Mayo:

Ingredients:

- 1/2 cup mayonnaise
- 2 tablespoons Sriracha sauce
- 1 teaspoon lime juice
- 1 teaspoon honey (optional, for sweetness)
- Salt to taste

Instructions:

1. In a bowl, combine mayonnaise and Sriracha sauce.
2. Add lime juice and honey (if using) to the bowl.

3. Mix the ingredients thoroughly until the Sriracha is evenly distributed.

4. Taste the Sriracha Mayo and add salt if needed.

5. Adjust the flavor by adding more Sriracha for extra heat or honey for sweetness, according to your preference.

6. Cover the bowl and refrigerate the Sriracha Mayo for at least 30 minutes before serving to allow the flavors to meld.

7. Serve the Sriracha Mayo as a spicy and tangy dipping sauce, or use it as a zesty spread for sandwiches, burgers, or wraps.

Tahini Sauce:

Ingredients:

- 1/2 cup tahini (sesame seed paste)
- 1/4 cup water
- 2 tablespoons olive oil
- 2 tablespoons lemon juice
- 1 clove garlic, minced
- 1/2 teaspoon ground cumin
- Salt to taste
- Optional: chopped fresh parsley for garnish

Instructions:

1. In a bowl, whisk together tahini, water, olive oil, and lemon juice.

2. Add minced garlic and ground cumin to the bowl.

3. Whisk the ingredients thoroughly until the tahini sauce is smooth and well combined.

4. Season the Tahini Sauce with salt to taste.

5. Taste and adjust the flavor by adding more lemon juice, garlic, cumin, or salt according to your preference.

6. If the sauce is too thick, you can add more water to reach your desired consistency.

7. Optionally, garnish with chopped fresh parsley for a burst of freshness.

8. Cover the bowl and let the Tahini Sauce sit for at least 30 minutes before serving to allow the flavors to meld.

Chimichurri Sauce:

Ingredients:

- 1 cup fresh parsley, finely chopped
- 1/4 cup fresh cilantro, finely chopped
- 3 cloves garlic, minced
- 1/2 cup extra virgin olive oil
- 2 tablespoons red wine vinegar
- 1 tablespoon lemon juice
- 1 teaspoon dried oregano
- 1/2 teaspoon red pepper flakes (adjust to taste)
- Salt and black pepper to taste

Instructions:

1. In a bowl, combine finely chopped parsley, finely chopped cilantro, and minced garlic.
2. Add extra virgin olive oil, red wine vinegar, and lemon juice to the bowl.
3. Mix the ingredients thoroughly until well combined.
4. Stir in dried oregano and red pepper flakes.
5. Season the Chimichurri Sauce with salt and black pepper to taste.
6. Taste and adjust the flavor by adding more vinegar, lemon juice, or seasoning according to your preference.
7. Allow the Chimichurri Sauce to sit for at least 15-30 minutes before serving to allow the flavors to meld.
8. Serve this vibrant and herby Chimichurri Sauce as a condiment for grilled meats, seafood, or roasted vegetables.

Tomatillo Salsa Verde:

Ingredients:

- 1 pound tomatillos, husked and washed
- 1/2 cup chopped onion
- 2 cloves garlic, minced
- 1-2 jalapeño peppers, seeded and chopped
- 1/2 cup fresh cilantro, chopped
- 1 tablespoon lime juice
- Salt to taste

Instructions:

1. Preheat the broiler in your oven.
2. Place the husked and washed tomatillos on a baking sheet and broil for about 5-7 minutes or until they start to char and soften.
3. In a blender or food processor, combine the broiled tomatillos, chopped onion, minced garlic, chopped jalapeño peppers, chopped cilantro, and lime juice.
4. Blend until the mixture reaches your desired salsa consistency.
5. Taste the Tomatillo Salsa Verde and add salt as needed.
6. Adjust the flavor by adding more lime juice, jalapeño, or cilantro according to your preference.
7. Allow the salsa to cool in the refrigerator for at least 30 minutes before serving to enhance the flavors.

Dressing Recipes:

Balsamic Vinaigrette:

Ingredients:

- 1/4 cup balsamic vinegar
- 1/2 cup extra virgin olive oil
- 1 tablespoon Dijon mustard

- 1 clove garlic, minced
- 1 teaspoon honey or maple syrup (optional, for sweetness)
- Salt and black pepper to taste

Instructions:

1. In a bowl, whisk together balsamic vinegar, extra virgin olive oil, Dijon mustard, and minced garlic.
2. If desired, add honey or maple syrup for a touch of sweetness.
3. Whisk the ingredients thoroughly until the vinaigrette is well combined.
4. Season the Balsamic Vinaigrette with salt and black pepper to taste.
5. Taste and adjust the flavor by adding more mustard, honey, or seasoning according to your preference.
6. Let the vinaigrette sit for at least 15 minutes before using to allow the flavors to meld.
7. Whisk again before drizzling over salads or using as a marinade for grilled vegetables or meats.

Lemon Tahini Dressing:

Ingredients:

- 1/3 cup tahini
- 1/4 cup water
- 3 tablespoons lemon juice
- 2 tablespoons extra virgin olive oil
- 1 clove garlic, minced
- 1 teaspoon honey or maple syrup
- Salt and black pepper to taste

Instructions:

1. In a bowl, whisk together tahini, water, lemon juice, and extra virgin olive oil.
2. Add minced garlic and honey (or maple syrup) to the bowl.
3. Whisk the ingredients thoroughly until the dressing is smooth and well combined.

4. Season the Lemon Tahini Dressing with salt and black pepper to taste.

5. Taste and adjust the flavor by adding more lemon juice, honey, or seasoning according to your preference.

6. If the dressing is too thick, you can add more water to reach your desired consistency.

7. Let the dressing sit for at least 15 minutes before serving to allow the flavors to meld.

8. Drizzle the Lemon Tahini Dressing over salads, roasted vegetables, or use as a dip for falafel.

Greek Yogurt Ranch Dressing:

Ingredients:

- 1 cup Greek yogurt
- 2 tablespoons mayonnaise
- 2 tablespoons chopped fresh dill
- 1 tablespoon chopped fresh chives
- 1 clove garlic, minced
- 1 tablespoon lemon juice
- 1/2 teaspoon onion powder
- Salt and black pepper to taste

Instructions:

1. In a bowl, combine Greek yogurt, mayonnaise, chopped fresh dill, chopped fresh chives, and minced garlic.

2. Add lemon juice and onion powder to the bowl.

3. Mix the ingredients thoroughly until the dressing is smooth and well combined.

4. Season the Greek Yogurt Ranch Dressing with salt and black pepper to taste.

5. Taste and adjust the flavor by adding more lemon juice, dill, chives, or seasoning according to your preference.

6. Refrigerate the dressing for at least 30 minutes before serving to allow the flavors to meld.

7. Serve the Greek Yogurt Ranch Dressing as a healthier alternative to traditional ranch dressing for salads, veggies, or as a dip.

Maple Dijon Dressing:

Ingredients:

- 1/4 cup Dijon mustard
- 2 tablespoons maple syrup
- 2 tablespoons apple cider vinegar
- 1/4 cup extra virgin olive oil
- 1 clove garlic, minced
- Salt and black pepper to taste

Instructions:

1. In a bowl, whisk together Dijon mustard, maple syrup, and apple cider vinegar.

2. Slowly drizzle in the extra virgin olive oil while continuously whisking to emulsify the dressing.

3. Add minced garlic to the bowl and whisk until the dressing is well combined.

4. Season the Maple Dijon Dressing with salt and black pepper to taste.

5. Taste and adjust the flavor by adding more maple syrup, Dijon mustard, or seasoning according to your preference.

6. Let the dressing sit for at least 15 minutes before serving to allow the flavors to meld.

7. Drizzle the Maple Dijon Dressing over salads, roasted vegetables, or use as a marinade for grilled chicken.

Cilantro Lime Dressing:

Ingredients:

- 1/2 cup fresh cilantro, chopped

- 1/4 cup lime juice
- 1/4 cup extra virgin olive oil
- 1 clove garlic, minced
- 1 teaspoon honey or maple syrup
- Salt and black pepper to taste

Instructions:

1. In a blender or food processor, combine chopped cilantro, lime juice, and minced garlic.
2. Blend until the cilantro is finely chopped.
3. With the blender running, slowly drizzle in the extra virgin olive oil until the mixture is smooth.
4. Add honey (or maple syrup) to the blender and blend again until well combined.
5. Season the Cilantro Lime Dressing with salt and black pepper to taste.
6. Taste and adjust the flavor by adding more lime juice, honey, or seasoning according to your preference.
7. Let the dressing sit for at least 15 minutes before serving to allow the flavors to meld.
8. Drizzle the Cilantro Lime Dressing over salads, grilled chicken, or use as a marinade for seafood.

Honey Mustard Vinaigrette:

Ingredients:

- 3 tablespoons Dijon mustard
- 2 tablespoons honey
- 2 tablespoons white wine vinegar
- 1/4 cup extra virgin olive oil
- 1 clove garlic, minced
- Salt and black pepper to taste

Instructions:

1. In a bowl, whisk together Dijon mustard, honey, and white wine vinegar.

2. Slowly drizzle in the extra virgin olive oil while continuously whisking to emulsify the vinaigrette.

3. Add minced garlic to the bowl and whisk until the vinaigrette is well combined.

4. Season the Honey Mustard Vinaigrette with salt and black pepper to taste.

5. Taste and adjust the flavor by adding more honey, Dijon mustard, or seasoning according to your preference.

6. Let the vinaigrette sit for at least 15 minutes before serving to allow the flavors to meld.

7. Drizzle the Honey Mustard Vinaigrette over salads, grilled vegetables, or use as a marinade for chicken.

Mango Avocado Lime Dressing:

Ingredients:

- 1 ripe mango, peeled and diced
- 1 ripe avocado, peeled and pitted
- 1/4 cup lime juice
- 2 tablespoons extra virgin olive oil
- 1 tablespoon honey or maple syrup
- 1 clove garlic, minced
- Salt and black pepper to taste

Instructions:

1. In a blender or food processor, combine diced mango, peeled and pitted avocado, lime juice, and minced garlic.

2. Blend until the mixture is smooth and creamy.

3. While the blender is running, slowly drizzle in the extra virgin olive oil until the dressing is well combined.

4. Add honey (or maple syrup) to the blender and blend again until the sweetness is evenly distributed.

5. Season the Mango Avocado Lime Dressing with salt and black pepper to taste.

6. Taste and adjust the flavor by adding more lime juice, honey, or seasoning according to your preference.

7. Let the dressing sit for at least 15 minutes before serving to allow the flavors to meld.

8. Drizzle the Mango Avocado Lime Dressing over salads, grilled chicken, or use as a refreshing dip.

Tahini Caesar Dressing:

Ingredients:

- 1/4 cup tahini
- 2 tablespoons lemon juice
- 2 tablespoons grated Parmesan cheese
- 1 tablespoon Dijon mustard
- 1 clove garlic, minced
- 1/4 cup extra virgin olive oil
- Salt and black pepper to taste

Instructions:

1. In a bowl, whisk together tahini, lemon juice, grated Parmesan cheese, Dijon mustard, and minced garlic.

2. Slowly drizzle in the extra virgin olive oil while continuously whisking to emulsify the dressing.

3. Season the Tahini Caesar Dressing with salt and black pepper to taste.

4. Taste and adjust the flavor by adding more lemon juice, Parmesan cheese, or seasoning according to your preference.

5. Let the dressing sit for at least 15 minutes before serving to allow the flavors to meld.

6. Drizzle the Tahini Caesar Dressing over romaine lettuce or your favorite salad ingredients.

Asian Sesame Ginger Dressing:

Ingredients:

- 3 tablespoons soy sauce
- 2 tablespoons rice vinegar
- 1 tablespoon sesame oil
- 1 tablespoon honey or maple syrup
- 1 tablespoon fresh ginger, grated
- 1 clove garlic, minced
- 2 tablespoons neutral-flavored oil (such as vegetable or grapeseed oil)
- 1 teaspoon sesame seeds
- Salt and black pepper to taste

Instructions:

1. In a bowl, whisk together soy sauce, rice vinegar, sesame oil, honey (or maple syrup), grated fresh ginger, and minced garlic.
2. Slowly drizzle in the neutral-flavored oil while continuously whisking to emulsify the dressing.
3. Add sesame seeds to the bowl and mix until well combined.
4. Season the Asian Sesame Ginger Dressing with salt and black pepper to taste.
5. Taste and adjust the flavor by adding more soy sauce, honey, or seasoning according to your preference.
6. Let the dressing sit for at least 15 minutes before serving to allow the flavors to meld.
7. Drizzle the Asian Sesame Ginger Dressing over mixed greens, Asian-inspired salads, or use as a marinade for grilled chicken or tofu.

Raspberry Walnut Vinaigrette:

Ingredients:

- 1/2 cup fresh or frozen raspberries
- 2 tablespoons red wine vinegar

- 1/4 cup extra virgin olive oil
- 1 tablespoon honey or maple syrup
- 1/4 cup chopped walnuts
- 1 teaspoon Dijon mustard
- Salt and black pepper to taste

Instructions:

1. In a blender or food processor, combine raspberries, red wine vinegar, and honey (or maple syrup).
2. Blend until the raspberries are pureed.
3. While the blender is running, slowly drizzle in the extra virgin olive oil until the mixture is smooth.
4. Add chopped walnuts and Dijon mustard to the blender and blend again until well combined.
5. Season the Raspberry Walnut Vinaigrette with salt and black pepper to taste.
6. Taste and adjust the flavor by adding more honey, vinegar, or seasoning according to your preference.
7. Let the vinaigrette sit for at least 15 minutes before serving to allow the flavors to meld.
8. Drizzle the Raspberry Walnut Vinaigrette over mixed greens, spinach, or use as a dressing for fruit salads.

Cranberry Orange Vinaigrette:

Ingredients:

- 1/2 cup fresh or frozen cranberries
- 1/4 cup orange juice
- 2 tablespoons white wine vinegar
- 1/4 cup extra virgin olive oil
- 2 tablespoons honey or maple syrup
- 1 teaspoon Dijon mustard

- 1/2 teaspoon orange zest
- Salt and black pepper to taste

Instructions:

1. In a blender or food processor, combine cranberries, orange juice, white wine vinegar, and honey (or maple syrup).
2. Blend until the cranberries are pureed.
3. While the blender is running, slowly drizzle in the extra virgin olive oil until the mixture is smooth.
4. Add Dijon mustard, orange zest, salt, and black pepper to the blender and blend again until well combined.
5. Season the Cranberry Orange Vinaigrette with additional salt, pepper, or sweetener to taste.
6. Let the vinaigrette sit for at least 15 minutes before serving to allow the flavors to meld.
7. Drizzle the Cranberry Orange Vinaigrette over mixed greens, spinach, or use as a dressing for fruit salads.

Sauce Recipes:

Homemade Marinara Sauce:

Ingredients:

- 2 tablespoons olive oil
- 1 onion, finely chopped
- 3 cloves garlic, minced
- 1 can (28 ounces) crushed tomatoes
- 1 can (14 ounces) diced tomatoes
- 1 teaspoon dried oregano
- 1 teaspoon dried basil
- 1/2 teaspoon dried thyme

- 1/2 teaspoon red pepper flakes (optional, for heat)
- Salt and black pepper to taste
- 1 teaspoon sugar (optional, to balance acidity)
- 1/4 cup fresh basil, chopped (optional, for added freshness)

Instructions:

1. In a large saucepan, heat olive oil over medium heat. Add finely chopped onion and sauté until softened, about 5 minutes.
2. Add minced garlic to the saucepan and sauté for an additional 1-2 minutes until fragrant.
3. Pour in the crushed tomatoes and diced tomatoes (with their juices) into the saucepan.
4. Stir in dried oregano, dried basil, dried thyme, red pepper flakes (if using), salt, and black pepper.
5. Optionally, add sugar to balance acidity. Stir the ingredients well.
6. Bring the marinara sauce to a simmer, then reduce the heat to low. Let it simmer uncovered for at least 30 minutes to allow the flavors to meld and the sauce to thicken.
7. Taste and adjust the seasoning as needed. If desired, stir in fresh chopped basil for added freshness.
8. Use the Homemade Marinara Sauce immediately or let it cool before storing in airtight containers in the refrigerator.

Creamy Alfredo Sauce:

Ingredients:

- 1/2 cup unsalted butter
- 2 cloves garlic, minced
- 2 cups heavy cream
- 1 cup grated Parmesan cheese
- 1 cup grated mozzarella cheese

- Salt and black pepper to taste
- 1/4 teaspoon ground nutmeg (optional, for a subtle warmth)
- Fresh parsley, chopped, for garnish (optional)

Instructions:

1. In a large saucepan, melt the unsalted butter over medium heat.
2. Add minced garlic to the melted butter and sauté for about 1-2 minutes until fragrant but not browned.
3. Pour in the heavy cream and bring it to a gentle simmer, stirring constantly.
4. Reduce the heat to low, then gradually whisk in the grated Parmesan and mozzarella cheeses until smooth and creamy.
5. Season the Creamy Alfredo Sauce with salt and black pepper to taste. Add ground nutmeg if desired for a subtle warmth.
6. Continue to stir the sauce over low heat until the cheese is fully melted and the sauce has reached your desired consistency.
7. Once the sauce is creamy and well combined, remove it from heat.
8. Serve the Creamy Alfredo Sauce immediately over your favorite pasta, or use it as a sauce for pizza, vegetables, or other dishes.

Teriyaki Glaze:

Ingredients:

- 1/2 cup soy sauce
- 1/4 cup water
- 2 tablespoons brown sugar
- 1 tablespoon honey
- 1 tablespoon rice vinegar
- 1 teaspoon grated fresh ginger
- 1 teaspoon minced garlic
- 1 tablespoon cornstarch (optional, for thickening)

Instructions:

1. In a small saucepan, combine soy sauce, water, brown sugar, honey, rice vinegar, grated fresh ginger, and minced garlic.

2. If you prefer a thicker glaze, mix cornstarch with a small amount of water to create a slurry. Stir the slurry into the saucepan.

3. Place the saucepan over medium heat and bring the mixture to a simmer, stirring constantly.

4. Allow the Teriyaki Glaze to simmer for 3-5 minutes or until it thickens to your desired consistency.

5. Taste the glaze and adjust the sweetness or saltiness by adding more honey or soy sauce if needed.

6. Remove the saucepan from heat and let the Teriyaki Glaze cool slightly before using.

7. Use the glaze as a marinade, basting sauce, or drizzle it over grilled meats, vegetables, or stir-fried dishes.

Honey Garlic Glaze:

Ingredients:

- 1/2 cup honey
- 1/4 cup soy sauce
- 2 cloves garlic, minced
- 1 tablespoon rice vinegar
- 1 teaspoon sesame oil (optional, for added flavor)
- 1 tablespoon cornstarch (optional, for thickening)

Instructions:

1. In a small saucepan, combine honey, soy sauce, minced garlic, rice vinegar, and sesame oil (if using).

2. If you prefer a thicker glaze, mix cornstarch with a small amount of water to create a slurry. Stir the slurry into the saucepan.

3. Place the saucepan over medium heat and bring the mixture to a simmer, stirring constantly.

4. Allow the Honey Garlic Glaze to simmer for 3-5 minutes or until it thickens to your desired consistency.

5. Taste the glaze and adjust the sweetness or saltiness by adding more honey or soy sauce if needed.

6. Remove the saucepan from heat and let the Honey Garlic Glaze cool slightly before using.

7. Use the glaze as a marinade, basting sauce, or drizzle it over grilled meats, chicken wings, or stir-fried dishes.

Cherry Balsamic Reduction:

Ingredients:

- 1 cup fresh or frozen cherries, pitted and halved
- 1/2 cup balsamic vinegar
- 2 tablespoons honey or maple syrup
- 1/4 teaspoon vanilla extract (optional)
- Pinch of salt

Instructions:

1. In a saucepan, combine cherries, balsamic vinegar, honey (or maple syrup), vanilla extract (if using), and a pinch of salt.

2. Place the saucepan over medium heat and bring the mixture to a simmer.

3. Reduce the heat to low and let the Cherry Balsamic Reduction simmer for 15-20 minutes or until the cherries have softened and the mixture has thickened.

4. Occasionally stir the reduction to prevent sticking and ensure even cooking.

5. Once the reduction has reached your desired consistency, remove the saucepan from heat.

6. Allow the Cherry Balsamic Reduction to cool slightly before using.

7. Strain the reduction through a fine mesh sieve to remove the cherry solids, or leave it as is for a chunkier texture.

8. Use the reduction as a drizzle over salads, grilled meats, desserts, or as a glaze for roasted vegetables.

Spicy Thai Peanut Sauce:

Ingredients:

- 1/2 cup peanut butter (smooth or chunky)
- 3 tablespoons soy sauce
- 2 tablespoons rice vinegar
- 1 tablespoon sesame oil
- 1 tablespoon honey or maple syrup
- 1 teaspoon grated fresh ginger
- 1 clove garlic, minced
- 1 teaspoon sriracha or chili garlic sauce (adjust to taste)
- 2 tablespoons water (adjust for desired consistency)
- Optional: chopped peanuts and chopped cilantro for garnish

Instructions:

1. In a bowl, whisk together peanut butter, soy sauce, rice vinegar, sesame oil, honey (or maple syrup), grated ginger, minced garlic, and sriracha.

2. Add water gradually, stirring continuously, until the Spicy Thai Peanut Sauce reaches your desired consistency.

3. Taste the sauce and adjust the sweetness, saltiness, or spiciness by adding more honey, soy sauce, or sriracha as needed.

4. Optionally, garnish the sauce with chopped peanuts and cilantro for added texture and freshness.

5. Use the Spicy Thai Peanut Sauce as a dipping sauce, dressing for salads, or drizzle it over noodles, stir-fries, or grilled meats.

Cajun Remoulade:

Ingredients:

- 1 cup mayonnaise
- 2 tablespoons Dijon mustard
- 2 tablespoons whole grain mustard
- 1 tablespoon hot sauce (adjust to taste)
- 1 tablespoon Worcestershire sauce
- 1 clove garlic, minced
- 1 tablespoon capers, drained and chopped
- 2 green onions, finely chopped
- 1 tablespoon fresh parsley, chopped
- 1 teaspoon Cajun seasoning
- Salt and black pepper to taste
- Lemon juice (optional, for extra tang)

Instructions:

1. In a bowl, combine mayonnaise, Dijon mustard, whole grain mustard, hot sauce, Worcestershire sauce, minced garlic, capers, chopped green onions, and chopped parsley.
2. Mix in Cajun seasoning, salt, and black pepper to taste.
3. If desired, add a squeeze of lemon juice for extra tanginess.
4. Taste the Cajun Remoulade and adjust the seasonings or heat level according to your preference.
5. Refrigerate the remoulade for at least 30 minutes before serving to allow the flavors to meld.
6. Serve the Cajun Remoulade as a dipping sauce for seafood, a spread for sandwiches, or as a flavorful accompaniment to various dishes.

Lemon Herb Butter Sauce:

Ingredients:

- 1/2 cup unsalted butter, softened
- Zest of 1 lemon
- 2 tablespoons fresh lemon juice
- 1 tablespoon fresh parsley, finely chopped
- 1 tablespoon fresh chives, finely chopped
- 1 teaspoon fresh thyme leaves
- Salt and black pepper to taste

Instructions:

1. In a bowl, combine softened unsalted butter, lemon zest, fresh lemon juice, finely chopped parsley, finely chopped chives, and fresh thyme leaves.
2. Mix the ingredients thoroughly until the herbs and lemon are evenly distributed throughout the butter.
3. Season the Lemon Herb Butter Sauce with salt and black pepper to taste.
4. Taste the sauce and adjust the lemon or herb flavors as needed.
5. You can use the Lemon Herb Butter Sauce immediately, or shape it into a log using plastic wrap and refrigerate for later use.
6. Slice the chilled butter log into rounds to top grilled meats, seafood, or vegetables just before serving.

Chimichurri Mayo:

Ingredients:

- 1 cup mayonnaise
- 1/4 cup fresh parsley, finely chopped
- 2 tablespoons fresh cilantro, finely chopped
- 2 cloves garlic, minced
- 2 tablespoons red wine vinegar
- 1 teaspoon dried oregano
- 1/2 teaspoon red pepper flakes (adjust to taste)
- Salt and black pepper to taste

- 1/4 cup extra virgin olive oil

Instructions:

1. In a bowl, combine mayonnaise, finely chopped fresh parsley, finely chopped fresh cilantro, minced garlic, red wine vinegar, dried oregano, and red pepper flakes.

2. Mix the ingredients thoroughly until the herbs and garlic are evenly distributed throughout the mayonnaise.

3. Season the Chimichurri Mayo with salt and black pepper to taste.

4. Slowly drizzle in the extra virgin olive oil while continuously whisking to incorporate it into the mayo mixture.

5. Taste the Chimichurri Mayo and adjust the seasonings or spice level according to your preference.

6. Refrigerate the Chimichurri Mayo for at least 30 minutes before serving to allow the flavors to meld.

7. Use the sauce as a zesty and herby condiment for sandwiches, burgers, or as a dipping sauce for fries.

Red Curry Coconut Sauce:

Ingredients:

- 1 can (14 ounces) coconut milk
- 2 tablespoons red curry paste
- 2 tablespoons soy sauce
- 1 tablespoon brown sugar
- 1 tablespoon lime juice
- 2 cloves garlic, minced
- 1 teaspoon grated fresh ginger
- 1 tablespoon vegetable oil
- 1 teaspoon sesame oil (optional, for added flavor)
- 1 tablespoon chopped cilantro (optional, for garnish)

- Salt to taste

Instructions:

1. In a saucepan, heat vegetable oil over medium heat. Add minced garlic and grated fresh ginger, sautéing for 1-2 minutes until fragrant.
2. Add red curry paste to the saucepan and stir, allowing it to cook for another 1-2 minutes.
3. Pour in coconut milk, soy sauce, brown sugar, and lime juice. Stir well to combine.
4. Bring the Red Curry Coconut Sauce to a simmer, then reduce the heat to low and let it simmer for 5-7 minutes to allow the flavors to meld and the sauce to thicken slightly.
5. If using, stir in sesame oil for added flavor.
6. Taste the sauce and adjust the sweetness or saltiness by adding more brown sugar or soy sauce if needed. Add salt to taste.
7. Optional: Garnish the Red Curry Coconut Sauce with chopped cilantro before serving.
8. Serve the sauce over rice, noodles, grilled meats, or vegetables.

Miso Ginger Glaze:

Ingredients:

- 1/4 cup white miso paste
- 2 tablespoons rice vinegar
- 1 tablespoon soy sauce
- 1 tablespoon honey or maple syrup
- 1 tablespoon fresh ginger, grated
- 1 clove garlic, minced
- 2 tablespoons sesame oil
- 1 tablespoon water (adjust for desired consistency)
- Optional: Sesame seeds and sliced green onions for garnish

Instructions:

1. In a bowl, whisk together white miso paste, rice vinegar, soy sauce, honey (or maple syrup), grated fresh ginger, and minced garlic.

2. Slowly drizzle in sesame oil while continuously whisking to incorporate it into the glaze.

3. Add water gradually to achieve the desired consistency, stirring well.

4. Taste the Miso Ginger Glaze and adjust the sweetness or saltiness by adding more honey or soy sauce if needed.

5. Optionally, garnish the glaze with sesame seeds and sliced green onions for added texture and freshness.

6. Use the Miso Ginger Glaze immediately as a marinade, basting sauce, or drizzle it over grilled meats, seafood, or vegetables.

CHAPTER 10: WEEKLY MEAL PLAN FOR PSORIASIS

Day 1:

Breakfast: Quinoa Breakfast Bowl with Berries and Nuts

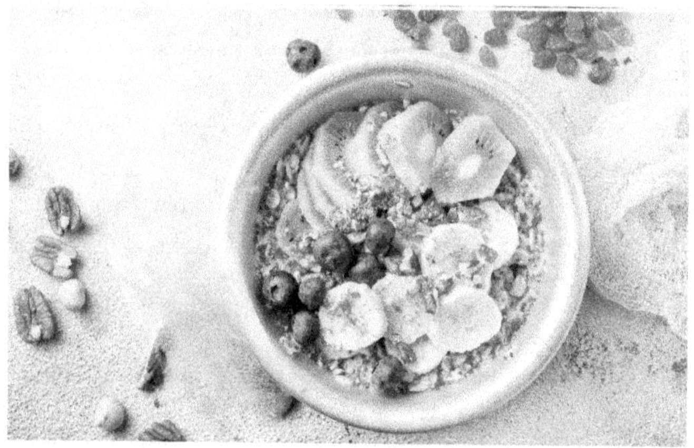

Ingredients:

- 1 cup quinoa, rinsed
- 2 cups water
- 1 cup mixed berries (blueberries, strawberries, raspberries)
- 1/4 cup chopped nuts (almonds, walnuts, or pistachios)
- 2 tablespoons chia seeds
- 1 tablespoon flaxseed meal
- 1 tablespoon honey or maple syrup (optional, for sweetness)
- 1/2 teaspoon cinnamon
- 1/2 cup almond milk or any non-dairy milk
- Fresh mint leaves for garnish (optional)

Instructions:

- In a medium saucepan, combine the rinsed quinoa and water. Bring to a boil, then reduce heat, cover, and simmer for 15-20 minutes or until the quinoa is cooked and water is absorbed.
- While the quinoa is cooking, prepare the berries by washing them and cutting larger berries into bite-sized pieces.
- Once the quinoa is cooked, fluff it with a fork and let it cool for a few minutes.
- In a serving bowl, combine the cooked quinoa, mixed berries, chopped nuts, chia seeds, flaxseed meal, and cinnamon.
- Drizzle honey or maple syrup over the mixture if you desire additional sweetness.
- Pour almond milk over the bowl, and gently stir to combine all the ingredients.
- Garnish with fresh mint leaves if you like.
- Serve the quinoa breakfast bowl immediately.

Lunch: Mediterranean Chickpea Bowl

Ingredients:

- 1 cup cooked quinoa or couscous
- 1 can (15 oz) chickpeas, drained and rinsed
- 1 cup cherry tomatoes, halved
- 1 cucumber, diced
- 1/2 red onion, finely chopped
- 1/4 cup Kalamata olives, sliced
- 1/4 cup feta cheese, crumbled
- 2 tablespoons extra-virgin olive oil
- 1 tablespoon balsamic vinegar
- 1 teaspoon dried oregano
- Salt and pepper to taste
- Fresh parsley for garnish

Instructions:

- In a large mixing bowl, combine the cooked quinoa or couscous, chickpeas, cherry tomatoes, cucumber, red onion, Kalamata olives, and feta cheese.
- In a small bowl, whisk together the extra-virgin olive oil, balsamic vinegar, dried oregano, salt, and pepper to create the dressing.
- Pour the dressing over the ingredients in the large bowl and toss gently to coat everything evenly.
- Taste and adjust seasoning if needed.
- Divide the Mediterranean chickpea mixture into individual serving bowls.
- Garnish each bowl with fresh parsley.
- Serve the Mediterranean Chickpea Bowl at room temperature or slightly chilled.

Dinner: Baked Lemon Herb Cod with Quinoa and Vegetable Salad

Ingredients:

- 4 cod fillets
- 2 tablespoons olive oil
- 2 tablespoons fresh lemon juice
- 2 teaspoons dried thyme
- 1 teaspoon dried rosemary
- 1 teaspoon garlic powder
- Salt and pepper to taste
- 1 cup quinoa, rinsed
- 2 cups water
- 1 cup cherry tomatoes, halved
- 1 bell pepper, diced
- 1 cucumber, diced
- 1/4 cup red onion, finely chopped
- 2 tablespoons fresh parsley, chopped
- 2 tablespoons feta cheese, crumbled (optional)
- 2 tablespoons balsamic vinaigrette dressing

Instructions:

1. Preheat the oven to 400°F (200°C).
2. In a small bowl, mix olive oil, lemon juice, dried thyme, dried rosemary, garlic powder, salt, and pepper to create a marinade for the cod fillets.
3. Place the cod fillets in a baking dish and coat them evenly with the marinade. Allow them to marinate for at least 15 minutes.
4. While the cod is marinating, rinse the quinoa and cook it according to package instructions using 2 cups of water.
5. In a large mixing bowl, combine the cooked quinoa, cherry tomatoes, bell pepper, cucumber, red onion, and fresh parsley.
6. In a separate small bowl, whisk together the balsamic vinaigrette dressing.
7. Pour the dressing over the quinoa and vegetable mixture, tossing gently to combine.
8. Place the marinated cod fillets in the preheated oven and bake for approximately 15-20 minutes or until the fish flakes easily with a fork.
9. While the cod is baking, prepare the quinoa and vegetable salad.
10. Once the cod is done, serve it on a plate alongside a generous portion of the quinoa and vegetable salad.
11. Optionally, sprinkle crumbled feta cheese over the top for added flavor.

Day 2:

Breakfast: Spinach and Mushroom Omelette

Ingredients:

- 3 large eggs
- 1/4 cup milk (or non-dairy alternative)
- 1 cup fresh spinach, chopped
- 1/2 cup mushrooms, sliced
- 1/4 cup onion, finely chopped

- 1 clove garlic, minced
- 1 tablespoon olive oil
- Salt and pepper to taste
- Optional: 1/4 cup shredded cheese (cheddar, feta, or your choice)

Instructions:

- In a bowl, whisk together eggs and milk until well combined. Season with a pinch of salt and pepper.
- Heat olive oil in a non-stick skillet over medium heat.
- Add chopped onions and garlic to the skillet, sautéing until they become translucent.
- Add sliced mushrooms to the skillet and cook until they are tender.
- Add chopped spinach to the skillet and cook until wilted.
- Pour the whisked eggs over the sautéed vegetables in the skillet.
- Allow the eggs to set slightly at the edges, then gently lift the edges with a spatula to let uncooked eggs flow underneath.
- Once the omelette is mostly set but still slightly runny on top, sprinkle shredded cheese (if using) over one half of the omelette.
- Fold the other half of the omelette over the cheese, creating a half-moon shape.
- Cook for an additional minute or until the cheese melts, and the omelette is fully cooked.
- Slide the omelette onto a plate and season with additional salt and pepper if needed.
- Garnish with fresh herbs or a sprinkle of cheese if desired.

Lunch: Veggie Stir-Fry with Tofu over Brown Rice

Ingredients:

- 3 large eggs
- 1/4 cup milk (or non-dairy alternative)
- 1 cup fresh spinach, chopped

- 1/2 cup mushrooms, sliced
- 1/4 cup onion, finely chopped
- 1 clove garlic, minced
- 1 tablespoon olive oil
- Salt and pepper to taste
- Optional: 1/4 cup shredded cheese (cheddar, feta, or your choice)

Instructions:

- In a bowl, whisk together eggs and milk until well combined. Season with a pinch of salt and pepper.
- Heat olive oil in a non-stick skillet over medium heat.
- Add chopped onions and garlic to the skillet, sautéing until they become translucent.
- Add sliced mushrooms to the skillet and cook until they are tender.
- Add chopped spinach to the skillet and cook until wilted.
- Pour the whisked eggs over the sautéed vegetables in the skillet.
- Allow the eggs to set slightly at the edges, then gently lift the edges with a spatula to let uncooked eggs flow underneath.
- Once the omelette is mostly set but still slightly runny on top, sprinkle shredded cheese (if using) over one half of the omelette.
- Fold the other half of the omelette over the cheese, creating a half-moon shape.
- Cook for an additional minute or until the cheese melts, and the omelette is fully cooked.
- Slide the omelette onto a plate and season with additional salt and pepper if needed.
- Garnish with fresh herbs or a sprinkle of cheese if desired.

Dinner: Quinoa Stuffed Bell Peppers with a Side of Mixed Berry Sorbet

Ingredients for Quinoa Stuffed Bell Peppers:

- 4 bell peppers, halved and seeds removed

- 1 cup quinoa, rinsed
- 2 cups vegetable broth
- 1 can (15 oz) black beans, drained and rinsed
- 1 cup corn kernels (fresh or frozen)
- 1 cup diced tomatoes
- 1 cup diced zucchini
- 1/2 cup red onion, finely chopped
- 2 cloves garlic, minced
- 1 teaspoon ground cumin
- 1 teaspoon chili powder
- Salt and pepper to taste
- 1 cup shredded cheese (cheddar or Mexican blend)
- Fresh cilantro for garnish

Ingredients for Mixed Berry Sorbet:

- 2 cups mixed berries (strawberries, blueberries, raspberries)
- 1/4 cup honey or maple syrup
- 1 tablespoon lemon juice

Instructions for Quinoa Stuffed Bell Peppers:

1. Preheat the oven to 375°F (190°C).
2. In a medium saucepan, combine quinoa and vegetable broth. Bring to a boil, then reduce heat, cover, and simmer for 15-20 minutes or until quinoa is cooked and liquid is absorbed.
3. In a large mixing bowl, combine cooked quinoa, black beans, corn, diced tomatoes, zucchini, red onion, garlic, cumin, chili powder, salt, and pepper.
4. Stuff each bell pepper half with the quinoa mixture and place them in a baking dish.
5. Top each stuffed pepper with shredded cheese.
6. Cover the baking dish with foil and bake in the preheated oven for 25-30 minutes or until the peppers are tender.

7. Garnish with fresh cilantro before serving.

Instructions for Mixed Berry Sorbet:

1. In a blender, combine mixed berries, honey or maple syrup, and lemon juice.

2. Blend until smooth.

3. Pour the mixture into a shallow dish and freeze for at least 3-4 hours, stirring every hour to prevent ice crystals from forming.

4. Once the sorbet is firm, use a fork to fluff and serve.

Day 3:

Breakfast: Chia Seed Pudding with Almond Milk and Fresh Fruit

Ingredients:

- 1/4 cup chia seeds
- 1 cup almond milk (or any non-dairy milk)
- 1 tablespoon maple syrup or honey
- 1/2 teaspoon vanilla extract
- Fresh fruits (berries, sliced kiwi, mango, etc.) for topping
- Nuts or seeds (optional, for garnish)

Instructions:

- In a bowl, mix chia seeds, almond milk, maple syrup or honey, and vanilla extract. Stir well to combine.
- Cover the bowl and refrigerate the mixture for at least 3 hours or overnight. This allows the chia seeds to absorb the liquid and create a pudding-like consistency.
- After the chia pudding has set, give it a good stir to break up any clumps.
- Spoon the chia pudding into serving glasses or bowls.
- Top the chia pudding with an assortment of fresh fruits.
- Optionally, sprinkle nuts or seeds on top for added texture.
- Drizzle a little extra maple syrup or honey over the fruit if you desire additional sweetness.

- Serve the chia seed pudding immediately and enjoy a delicious and nutritious breakfast!

Lunch: Caprese Salad with Balsamic Glaze

Ingredients:

- 4 large ripe tomatoes, sliced
- 1 ball fresh mozzarella cheese, sliced
- Fresh basil leaves
- Extra-virgin olive oil
- Balsamic glaze
- Salt and pepper to taste

Instructions:

- Arrange the tomato and mozzarella slices on a serving platter, alternating them for a visually appealing presentation.
- Tuck fresh basil leaves between the tomato and mozzarella slices.
- Drizzle extra-virgin olive oil over the tomato and mozzarella slices.
- Season with salt and pepper to taste.
- Drizzle balsamic glaze over the top for a sweet and tangy finish.
- Optionally, garnish with additional fresh basil leaves.
- Serve the Caprese Salad immediately, and enjoy the classic combination of tomatoes, mozzarella, and basil with the delightful addition of balsamic glaze.

Dinner: Grilled Teriyaki Mahi-Mahi with Roasted Sweet Potato Wedges

Ingredients for Grilled Teriyaki Mahi-Mahi:

- 4 Mahi-Mahi fillets
- 1/2 cup soy sauce
- 1/4 cup mirin
- 2 tablespoons honey
- 1 tablespoon rice vinegar

- 1 teaspoon sesame oil

- 2 cloves garlic, minced

- 1 teaspoon fresh ginger, grated

- Sesame seeds for garnish (optional)

- Sliced green onions for garnish (optional)

Ingredients for Roasted Sweet Potato Wedges:

- 2 large sweet potatoes, peeled and cut into wedges

- 2 tablespoons olive oil

- 1 teaspoon smoked paprika

- 1 teaspoon garlic powder

- 1/2 teaspoon cayenne pepper (optional for spice)

- Salt and pepper to taste

Instructions for Grilled Teriyaki Mahi-Mahi:

1. In a bowl, whisk together soy sauce, mirin, honey, rice vinegar, sesame oil, minced garlic, and grated ginger to create the teriyaki marinade.

2. Place Mahi-Mahi fillets in a shallow dish and pour half of the teriyaki marinade over them. Reserve the remaining marinade for basting.

3. Marinate the Mahi-Mahi in the refrigerator for at least 30 minutes.

4. Preheat the grill to medium-high heat.

5. Grill the Mahi-Mahi fillets for 4-5 minutes per side or until cooked through, basting with the reserved teriyaki marinade during grilling.

6. Remove from the grill and garnish with sesame seeds and sliced green onions if desired.

Instructions for Roasted Sweet Potato Wedges:

1. Preheat the oven to 425°F (220°C).

2. In a large bowl, toss sweet potato wedges with olive oil, smoked paprika, garlic powder, cayenne pepper (if using), salt, and pepper until evenly coated.

3. Spread the sweet potato wedges in a single layer on a baking sheet.

4. Roast in the preheated oven for 25-30 minutes or until the sweet potatoes are golden brown and tender, flipping halfway through.

Day 4:

Breakfast: Greek Yogurt Parfait with Granola and Fresh Fruit

Ingredients:

- 1 cup Greek yogurt
- 1/2 cup granola
- 1 cup mixed fresh fruit (berries, sliced banana, kiwi, etc.)
- Honey or maple syrup for drizzling (optional)

Instructions:

- In a glass or bowl, layer half of the Greek yogurt at the bottom.
- Add a layer of half the granola on top of the yogurt.
- Place a portion of mixed fresh fruit over the granola layer.
- Repeat the layers with the remaining Greek yogurt, granola, and fresh fruit.
- Optionally, drizzle honey or maple syrup over the top for added sweetness.
- Serve the Greek Yogurt Parfait immediately and enjoy a wholesome and satisfying breakfast!

Lunch: Sweet Potato and Lentil Soup

Ingredients:

- 1 cup dried green or brown lentils, rinsed
- 2 large sweet potatoes, peeled and diced
- 1 onion, finely chopped
- 2 carrots, peeled and sliced
- 2 celery stalks, chopped
- 3 cloves garlic, minced
- 1 teaspoon ground cumin

- 1 teaspoon ground coriander
- 1/2 teaspoon smoked paprika
- 6 cups vegetable broth
- 1 can (14 oz) diced tomatoes, undrained
- 2 bay leaves
- Salt and pepper to taste
- 2 tablespoons olive oil
- Fresh cilantro or parsley for garnish (optional)

Instructions:

- In a large pot, heat olive oil over medium heat.
- Add chopped onions, carrots, and celery. Sauté until the vegetables are softened.
- Add minced garlic, ground cumin, ground coriander, and smoked paprika to the pot. Stir well to combine.
- Add sweet potatoes, lentils, vegetable broth, diced tomatoes (with their juices), and bay leaves to the pot.
- Bring the soup to a boil, then reduce heat to low, cover, and simmer for 25-30 minutes or until lentils and sweet potatoes are tender.
- Season the soup with salt and pepper to taste.
- Remove the bay leaves and discard them.
- Using an immersion blender, blend a portion of the soup to reach your desired consistency. Alternatively, transfer a portion to a blender and blend, then return it to the pot.
- Adjust seasoning if needed and let the soup simmer for an additional 5-10 minutes.
- Serve the Sweet Potato and Lentil Soup hot, garnished with fresh cilantro or parsley if desired.

Dinner: Zucchini Noodles with Pesto and a side of Lemon Garlic Butter Shrimp Scampi

Ingredients for Zucchini Noodles with Pesto:

- 4 medium-sized zucchini, spiralized into noodles
- 1 cup cherry tomatoes, halved
- 1/2 cup fresh basil leaves
- 1/3 cup pine nuts
- 1/2 cup grated Parmesan cheese
- 2 cloves garlic, minced
- 1/2 cup extra-virgin olive oil
- Salt and pepper to taste

Ingredients for Lemon Garlic Butter Shrimp Scampi:

- 1 pound large shrimp, peeled and deveined
- 4 tablespoons unsalted butter
- 4 cloves garlic, minced
- Zest of 1 lemon
- Juice of 1 lemon
- 1/4 cup fresh parsley, chopped
- Salt and pepper to taste

Instructions for Zucchini Noodles with Pesto:

1. In a blender or food processor, combine basil, pine nuts, Parmesan cheese, minced garlic, and a pinch of salt and pepper. Pulse until finely chopped.
2. With the blender or food processor running, slowly add the olive oil until the pesto reaches a smooth consistency. Adjust seasoning if needed.
3. In a large pan, heat a little olive oil over medium heat. Add zucchini noodles and cherry tomatoes, and sauté for 2-3 minutes or until the noodles are just tender.
4. Add the pesto to the zucchini noodles, tossing to coat evenly. Cook for an additional 1-2 minutes until heated through.
5. Serve the Zucchini Noodles with Pesto hot.

Instructions for Lemon Garlic Butter Shrimp Scampi:

1. In a large skillet, melt butter over medium heat.
2. Add minced garlic to the skillet and sauté for 1-2 minutes until fragrant.

3. Add shrimp to the skillet and cook for 2-3 minutes per side or until they turn pink and opaque.

4. Stir in lemon zest, lemon juice, chopped parsley, salt, and pepper. Cook for an additional 1-2 minutes.

5. Serve the Lemon Garlic Butter Shrimp Scampi hot, alongside the Zucchini Noodles with Pesto.

Day 5:

Breakfast: Banana Walnut Smoothie

Ingredients:

- 1 ripe banana, peeled and sliced
- 1/2 cup Greek yogurt
- 1/2 cup milk (dairy or non-dairy)
- 1/4 cup rolled oats
- 1/4 cup chopped walnuts
- 1 tablespoon honey or maple syrup (optional for sweetness)
- Ice cubes (optional)

Instructions:

- In a blender, combine sliced banana, Greek yogurt, milk, rolled oats, and chopped walnuts.
- Optionally, add honey or maple syrup for sweetness.
- If you prefer a colder smoothie, add a handful of ice cubes to the blender.
- Blend all the ingredients until smooth and creamy.
- Pour the Banana Walnut Smoothie into a glass.
- Garnish with additional chopped walnuts or banana slices if desired.
- Serve the smoothie immediately and enjoy a delicious and nutrient-packed breakfast!

Lunch: Chickpea and Spinach Quesadilla

Ingredients:

- 1 can (15 oz) chickpeas, drained and rinsed
- 2 cups fresh spinach, chopped
- 1 cup shredded cheese (cheddar, Monterey Jack, or your choice)
- 4 large whole wheat or corn tortillas
- 1/2 cup diced tomatoes
- 1/4 cup diced red onion
- 1 teaspoon ground cumin
- 1 teaspoon paprika
- 1/2 teaspoon garlic powder
- Salt and pepper to taste
- Olive oil for cooking
- Greek yogurt or salsa for serving (optional)

Instructions:

- In a large skillet, heat olive oil over medium heat.
- Add chickpeas to the skillet and sprinkle with ground cumin, paprika, garlic powder, salt, and pepper. Cook for 5-7 minutes, stirring occasionally, until chickpeas are lightly browned.
- Add chopped spinach to the skillet and cook until wilted.
- In a separate dry skillet, place a tortilla over medium heat.
- Sprinkle a portion of shredded cheese over half of the tortilla.
- Spoon a portion of the chickpea and spinach mixture over the cheese.
- Sprinkle diced tomatoes and red onions over the top.
- Fold the tortilla in half, creating a quesadilla, and press down gently with a spatula.
- Cook for 2-3 minutes on each side or until the tortilla is golden brown and the cheese is melted.

- Repeat the process for the remaining tortillas.
- Slice the quesadillas into wedges.
- Serve the Chickpea and Spinach Quesadilla warm, optionally with Greek yogurt or salsa on the side.

Dinner: Quinoa and Black Bean Stuffed Peppers with a side of Cucumber Tomato Salad

Ingredients for Quinoa and Black Bean Stuffed Peppers:

- 4 large bell peppers, halved and seeds removed
- 1 cup quinoa, rinsed
- 2 cups vegetable broth
- 1 can (15 oz) black beans, drained and rinsed
- 1 cup corn kernels (fresh or frozen)
- 1 cup diced tomatoes
- 1/2 cup red onion, finely chopped
- 2 cloves garlic, minced
- 1 teaspoon ground cumin
- 1 teaspoon chili powder
- Salt and pepper to taste
- 1 cup shredded cheese (cheddar or Mexican blend)
- Fresh cilantro for garnish (optional)
- Sour cream or Greek yogurt for serving (optional)

Ingredients for Cucumber Tomato Salad:

- 1 cucumber, diced
- 1 cup cherry tomatoes, halved
- 1/4 cup red onion, finely chopped
- 2 tablespoons fresh parsley, chopped
- 2 tablespoons olive oil
- 1 tablespoon red wine vinegar

- Salt and pepper to taste

Instructions for Quinoa and Black Bean Stuffed Peppers:

1. Preheat the oven to 375°F (190°C).
2. In a medium saucepan, combine quinoa and vegetable broth. Bring to a boil, then reduce heat, cover, and simmer for 15-20 minutes or until quinoa is cooked and liquid is absorbed.
3. In a large mixing bowl, combine cooked quinoa, black beans, corn, diced tomatoes, red onion, garlic, cumin, chili powder, salt, and pepper.
4. Stuff each bell pepper half with the quinoa mixture and place them in a baking dish.
5. Top each stuffed pepper with shredded cheese.
6. Cover the baking dish with foil and bake in the preheated oven for 25-30 minutes or until the peppers are tender.
7. Garnish with fresh cilantro before serving.

Instructions for Cucumber Tomato Salad:

1. In a bowl, combine diced cucumber, cherry tomatoes, red onion, and fresh parsley.
2. In a small bowl, whisk together olive oil, red wine vinegar, salt, and pepper.
3. Pour the dressing over the salad and toss gently to combine.

Day 6:

Breakfast: Buckwheat Pancakes with Blueberry Compote

Ingredients for Buckwheat Pancakes:

- 1 cup buckwheat flour
- 1 tablespoon sugar
- 1 teaspoon baking powder
- 1/2 teaspoon baking soda
- 1/4 teaspoon salt
- 1 cup buttermilk (or non-dairy milk with 1 tablespoon vinegar)

- 1 large egg
- 2 tablespoons melted butter (or oil)
- Cooking spray or additional butter for the pan

Ingredients for Blueberry Compote:

- 1 cup fresh or frozen blueberries
- 2 tablespoons maple syrup or honey
- 1 tablespoon lemon juice
- 1/2 teaspoon vanilla extract (optional)

Instructions for Buckwheat Pancakes:

1. In a large mixing bowl, whisk together buckwheat flour, sugar, baking powder, baking soda, and salt.
2. In a separate bowl, whisk together buttermilk, egg, and melted butter.
3. Pour the wet ingredients into the dry ingredients and stir until just combined. Do not overmix; a few lumps are okay.
4. Heat a griddle or non-stick skillet over medium heat. Lightly coat with cooking spray or butter.
5. Pour 1/4 cup portions of batter onto the griddle for each pancake.
6. Cook until bubbles form on the surface, then flip and cook until the other side is golden brown.
7. Repeat until all the batter is used.

Instructions for Blueberry Compote:

- In a small saucepan, combine blueberries, maple syrup or honey, lemon juice, and vanilla extract (if using).
- Bring the mixture to a simmer over medium heat.
- Cook for 5-7 minutes, stirring occasionally, until the blueberries burst and the compote thickens.
- Remove from heat and let it cool slightly.

Lunch: Shrimp and Mango Salad

Ingredients:

- 1 pound shrimp, peeled and deveined
- 2 tablespoons olive oil
- 1 teaspoon smoked paprika
- Salt and pepper to taste
- 4 cups mixed salad greens
- 1 ripe mango, peeled, pitted, and diced
- 1 cucumber, diced
- 1/4 cup red onion, thinly sliced
- 1/4 cup fresh cilantro, chopped

For the Lime Vinaigrette:

- 3 tablespoons olive oil
- 2 tablespoons lime juice
- 1 tablespoon honey
- 1 teaspoon Dijon mustard
- Salt and pepper to taste

Instructions:

- In a bowl, toss the shrimp with olive oil, smoked paprika, salt, and pepper until evenly coated.
- Heat a skillet over medium-high heat and cook the shrimp for 2-3 minutes per side or until they turn pink and opaque. Remove from heat and set aside.
- In a large salad bowl, combine mixed salad greens, diced mango, cucumber, red onion, and chopped cilantro.
- In a small bowl, whisk together olive oil, lime juice, honey, Dijon mustard, salt, and pepper to create the lime vinaigrette.
- Add the cooked shrimp to the salad bowl.
- Drizzle the lime vinaigrette over the salad and shrimp, tossing gently to coat everything.

- Serve the Shrimp and Mango Salad immediately and enjoy a refreshing and flavorful lunch!

Dinner: Eggplant and Chickpea Curry with Cauliflower Rice

Ingredients for Eggplant and Chickpea Curry:

- 1 large eggplant, diced
- 1 can (15 oz) chickpeas, drained and rinsed
- 1 onion, finely chopped
- 2 tomatoes, diced
- 3 cloves garlic, minced
- 1 tablespoon fresh ginger, grated
- 1 can (14 oz) coconut milk
- 2 tablespoons curry powder
- 1 teaspoon ground cumin
- 1 teaspoon ground coriander
- 1/2 teaspoon turmeric
- 1/2 teaspoon chili powder (adjust to taste)
- Salt and pepper to taste
- 2 tablespoons vegetable oil
- Fresh cilantro for garnish

Ingredients for Cauliflower Rice:

- 1 medium-sized cauliflower, grated or processed into rice-sized pieces
- 2 tablespoons olive oil
- Salt and pepper to taste

Instructions for Eggplant and Chickpea Curry:

1. Heat vegetable oil in a large skillet over medium heat.
2. Add chopped onions and sauté until softened.
3. Add minced garlic and grated ginger to the skillet. Sauté for an additional 1-2 minutes until fragrant.

4. Stir in curry powder, ground cumin, ground coriander, turmeric, and chili powder. Cook for 1-2 minutes to toast the spices.

5. Add diced eggplant to the skillet and cook until it starts to brown.

6. Pour in coconut milk, add diced tomatoes, and bring the mixture to a simmer.

7. Add chickpeas to the skillet, season with salt and pepper, and simmer for 15-20 minutes or until the eggplant is tender.

8. Adjust seasoning if needed and garnish with fresh cilantro.

Instructions for Cauliflower Rice:

1. In a separate pan, heat olive oil over medium heat.

2. Add grated cauliflower and sauté for 5-7 minutes or until the cauliflower is tender.

3. Season with salt and pepper to taste.

Day 7:

Breakfast: Oatmeal with Berries and Almonds

Ingredients:

- 1 cup old-fashioned oats
- 2 cups milk (dairy or non-dairy)
- 1 cup mixed berries (blueberries, strawberries, raspberries)
- 1/4 cup almonds, chopped
- 1 tablespoon honey or maple syrup (optional, for sweetness)
- 1/2 teaspoon vanilla extract
- Pinch of salt

Instructions:

- In a saucepan, combine oats, milk, and a pinch of salt.
- Bring the mixture to a simmer over medium heat, stirring occasionally.
- Once the oats begin to thicken, reduce the heat to low and continue to cook until the oats are creamy and fully cooked.
- Stir in vanilla extract and sweeten with honey or maple syrup if desired.

- In a serving bowl, spoon the cooked oatmeal.

- Top the oatmeal with mixed berries and chopped almonds.

- Optionally, drizzle a little extra honey or maple syrup over the top.

- Serve the Oatmeal with Berries and Almonds warm and enjoy a nutritious and satisfying breakfast!

Lunch: Grilled Chicken Caesar Salad

Ingredients:

- 2 boneless, skinless chicken breasts

- Salt and black pepper to taste

- 1 tablespoon olive oil

- 1 head romaine lettuce, washed and chopped

- 1 cup cherry tomatoes, halved

- 1/2 cup croutons

- 1/4 cup grated Parmesan cheese

For the Caesar Dressing:

- 1/2 cup mayonnaise

- 2 tablespoons grated Parmesan cheese

- 2 tablespoons lemon juice

- 1 tablespoon Dijon mustard

- 2 cloves garlic, minced

- 2 anchovy fillets, finely chopped (optional)

- Salt and black pepper to taste

Instructions:

- Preheat the grill or grill pan to medium-high heat.

- Season the chicken breasts with salt and black pepper.

- Brush the chicken breasts with olive oil.

- Grill the chicken for 6-8 minutes per side or until fully cooked (internal temperature of 165°F or 74°C). Allow the chicken to rest for a few minutes before slicing.
- In a bowl, whisk together mayonnaise, grated Parmesan, lemon juice, Dijon mustard, minced garlic, anchovies (if using), salt, and black pepper to create the Caesar dressing.
- In a large salad bowl, combine chopped romaine lettuce, cherry tomatoes, croutons, and grated Parmesan cheese.
- Slice the grilled chicken breasts and arrange them on top of the salad.
- Drizzle the Caesar dressing over the salad and chicken.
- Toss the salad gently to coat everything in the dressing.
- Serve the Grilled Chicken Caesar Salad immediately, and enjoy a flavorful and satisfying lunch!

Dinner: Spaghetti Squash Primavera with Grilled Asparagus

Ingredients:

- 1 medium-sized spaghetti squash
- 1 bunch asparagus, trimmed
- 2 tablespoons olive oil, divided
- 1 bell pepper, thinly sliced
- 1 zucchini, thinly sliced
- 1 carrot, julienned
- 2 cloves garlic, minced
- 1 cup cherry tomatoes, halved
- 1/4 cup fresh basil, chopped
- Salt and black pepper to taste
- Grated Parmesan cheese for serving (optional)

Instructions:

1. Preheat the oven to 400°F (200°C).

2. Cut the spaghetti squash in half lengthwise. Scoop out the seeds and fibers.

3. Rub the cut sides of the squash with 1 tablespoon of olive oil. Place the squash, cut side down, on a baking sheet.

4. Roast the spaghetti squash in the preheated oven for 40-50 minutes or until the flesh is tender and can be easily scraped with a fork.

5. While the squash is roasting, toss asparagus spears with 1 tablespoon of olive oil and season with salt and black pepper. Grill the asparagus on a grill pan or outdoor grill until tender and slightly charred. Set aside.

6. In a large skillet, heat olive oil over medium heat. Add sliced bell pepper, zucchini, and julienned carrot. Sauté until the vegetables are tender-crisp.

7. Add minced garlic to the skillet and cook for an additional 1-2 minutes until fragrant.

8. Stir in cherry tomatoes and chopped basil. Cook for 2-3 minutes until the tomatoes are slightly softened.

9. Using a fork, scrape the roasted spaghetti squash flesh into strands. Add the squash strands to the skillet with the sautéed vegetables.

10. Toss everything together until well combined. Season with additional salt and black pepper if needed.

11. Arrange the spaghetti squash primavera on serving plates and top with grilled asparagus.

12. Optionally, sprinkle grated Parmesan cheese over the top for added flavor.

Snacks:

Mixed Nuts

Ingredients:

- 1 cup almonds
- 1 cup walnuts
- 1 cup cashews

- 1 cup pecans
- 1 cup hazelnuts
- 1 tablespoon olive oil
- 1 tablespoon honey
- 1 teaspoon sea salt
- 1 teaspoon ground cinnamon (optional)

Instructions:

- Preheat the oven to 325°F (163°C).
- In a large bowl, combine almonds, walnuts, cashews, pecans, and hazelnuts.
- In a small saucepan, heat olive oil and honey over low heat until well combined.
- Pour the olive oil and honey mixture over the mixed nuts and toss to coat evenly.
- Spread the coated nuts in a single layer on a baking sheet lined with parchment paper.
- Sprinkle sea salt over the nuts. Optionally, add ground cinnamon for a hint of warmth and flavor.
- Bake in the preheated oven for 15-20 minutes, stirring once halfway through, until the nuts are golden brown and fragrant.
- Remove the mixed nuts from the oven and let them cool completely.
- Once cooled, break apart any clusters and store the mixed nuts in an airtight container.

Greek Yogurt with Honey

Ingredients:

- 1 cup Greek yogurt
- 2 tablespoons honey (adjust to taste)
- Fresh fruit (optional, for garnish)
- Nuts (optional, for garnish)

Instructions:

- Spoon Greek yogurt into a serving bowl.

- Drizzle honey over the Greek yogurt.

- Using a spoon or a spatula, gently swirl the honey into the yogurt to combine.

- Optionally, garnish with fresh fruit such as berries or sliced fruits.

- Optionally, sprinkle nuts like almonds or walnuts on top for added texture.

- Serve the Greek Yogurt with Honey immediately and enjoy a simple and delightful treat!

Fresh Fruit Slices

Ingredients:

- Assorted fresh fruits (e.g., watermelon, cantaloupe, pineapple, strawberries, kiwi, grapes)

- Fresh mint leaves for garnish (optional)

- Lime or lemon juice for drizzling (optional)

Instructions:

- Wash and prepare the fruits. Peel and slice larger fruits like watermelon, cantaloupe, and pineapple. Hull and slice strawberries. Peel and slice kiwi. Leave grapes whole or slice them in half.

- Arrange the sliced fruits on a serving platter or individual plates.

- Optionally, drizzle a little lime or lemon juice over the fruit slices for a refreshing citrus flavor.

- Garnish with fresh mint leaves for added freshness (optional).

- Serve the fresh fruit slices immediately and enjoy a vibrant and healthy snack or dessert!

Hummus with Veggie Sticks

Ingredients for Hummus:

- 1 can (15 oz) chickpeas, drained and rinsed

- 1/4 cup tahini

- 2 tablespoons olive oil

- 2 tablespoons lemon juice
- 2 cloves garlic, minced
- 1/2 teaspoon ground cumin
- Salt to taste
- Water (as needed for desired consistency)

Ingredients for Veggie Sticks:

- Carrot sticks
- Cucumber sticks
- Bell pepper strips
- Cherry tomatoes

Instructions for Hummus:

1. In a food processor, combine chickpeas, tahini, olive oil, lemon juice, minced garlic, ground cumin, and a pinch of salt.
2. Process the ingredients until smooth. If needed, add water gradually to achieve your desired hummus consistency.
3. Taste and adjust salt and lemon juice as necessary.
4. Transfer the hummus to a serving bowl.

Instructions for Veggie Sticks:

- Wash and prepare carrot sticks, cucumber sticks, bell pepper strips, and cherry tomatoes.
- Arrange the veggie sticks on a platter alongside the hummus.
- Serve the Hummus with Veggie Sticks immediately and enjoy a tasty and nutritious snack!

Rice Cakes with Avocado

Ingredients:

- Rice cakes (whole grain or plain)
- 1 ripe avocado
- Salt and black pepper to taste

- Red pepper flakes (optional, for spice)
- Lime or lemon wedges for garnish (optional)
- Fresh cilantro or parsley for garnish (optional)

Instructions:

1. Slice the avocado in half, remove the pit, and scoop out the flesh into a bowl.
2. Mash the avocado with a fork until it reaches your desired level of smoothness.
3. Season the mashed avocado with salt and black pepper. Optionally, add red pepper flakes for a touch of spice.
4. Spread a generous layer of the seasoned mashed avocado onto each rice cake.
5. Optionally, garnish with lime or lemon wedges for a citrusy kick.
6. Top with fresh cilantro or parsley for added freshness (optional).
7. Serve the Rice Cakes with Avocado immediately and enjoy a simple and tasty snack or light meal!

DINING OUT WITH PSORIASIS

1. In advance, look for restaurants that provide healthful and psoriasis-friendly options and check their menus online.
2. Communicate food Requirements: Do not be afraid to tell the server about your food preferences or limits. Many establishments are willing to meet specific requests.
3. Choose Grilled or Baked Options: Instead of frying, choose dishes that are grilled, baked or steamed. This can help regulate the inflammation associated with psoriasis.
4. Prioritize Whole Foods: To support general skin health, prioritize whole unprocessed foods such as lean meats, fruits and vegetables.
5. Be Wary of Condiments: Be wary of sauces and dressings as some may contain substances that cause inflammation. Request them on the side.
6. Control Portion Sizes: To keep your caloric intake under control, consider sharing dishes or opting for smaller servings.

7. Limit your alcohol consumption: Excessive alcohol consumption can aggravate psoriasis symptoms. Choose moderation or non-alcoholic substitutes.

8. Maintain Hydration: Water is essential for skin health. Choose water or herbal teas over sugary beverages to remain hydrated.

9. Mindful Eating entails eating deliberately and savoring each bite. This not only improves your dining experience but it also aids with portion control.

10. Choose Stress-Free Environments: To reduce stress, choose eateries with a relaxing ambiance. Stress has been shown to have an impact on psoriasis symptoms.

MAKING INFORMED MENU CHOICES

1. Review the Menu in Advance: Before you arrive at the restaurant, look over the menu online to give yourself time to consider healthier selections.

2. Balance Your Plate: Aim for a well-balanced dinner that includes a variety of lean proteins, complete grains, and veggies.

3. Mindful Portion Sizes: If you want to avoid overeating, consider sharing dishes or ordering smaller portions.

4. Request Modifications: Do not be afraid to request changes to accommodate your dietary choices or constraints. Most establishments are willing to work with you.

5. Inquire about Methods of Preparation: Inquire about how foods are prepared; choose grilled, roasted or steamed options over fried or excessively processed options.

6. Select Smart Starters: To help limit your hunger and add nutrients to your meal, start with a salad or broth-based soup.

7. Keep an eye out for hidden sugars: Be wary of hidden sugars in sauces, dressings and beverages. Choose foods with few added sugars.

8. Choose Lean Proteins: To support muscular health and overall well-being, choose lean protein sources such as grilled chicken, fish or lentils.

9. Include Colorful veggies: Include a variety of colorful veggies in your meal to ensure a wide range of nutrients and antioxidants.

10. Choose water or other low-calorie beverages over sugary drinks to hydrate wisely. Keeping hydrated benefits general health and can aid in portion control.

INCORPORATING EXERCISE INTO YOUR ROUTINE

1. Morning Rituals: Invigorate your body and mind by starting your day with a brisk walk, jog or a fast home workout.

2. Lunchtime Stretches: Take use of your lunch break to go for a little stroll, stretch or even do a small office workout to break up your sedentary day.

3. Commute Creatively: Walk or cycle to work if possible. If so, consider parking further away or exiting public transit a stop earlier to add extra steps.

4. Deskercise: Incorporate modest activities into your workday, such as stretches, leg lifts or seated exercises to keep you active during office hours.

5. Make physical activity a family affair. As a bonding activity, go for nighttime walks together, play sports or do home workouts.

6. TV Workout: Make the most of your TV time by combining exercises. During the commercial breaks of your favorite show, you can practice squats, lunges or yoga poses.

7. Stair Climbing: Whenever possible, choose stairs over lifts. It's an easy but effective approach to incorporate cardio into your everyday routine.

8. Weekend experiences: Make weekends active experiences by hiking, riding or discovering a new park. This can make exercise feel satisfying.

9. Socialise and Sweat: Get together with friends for activities that require mobility such as group fitness courses, dancing or playing sports.

10. Set Realistic Goals: Set achievable fitness goals and gradually incorporate them into your routine. Small, durable adjustments that are consistent frequently lead to long-term success.

CHAPTER 11: MANAGING STRESS FOR PSORIASIS RELIEF

1. Use Relaxation Techniques: To help manage stress, incorporate relaxation techniques such as deep breathing, meditation or yoga into your daily routine.
2. Regular Physical Activity: Exercise has been shown to lower stress and promote general well-being, benefitting both mental and skin health.
3. Establish a Sleep Routine: Maintain a consistent sleep schedule to prioritize quality sleep. A well-rested body is better able to handle stress.
4. Mindfulness & Meditation: Use mindfulness practices to be present in the moment, cultivate tranquilly and reduce stress.
5. Time Management: Plan your day ahead of time to avoid feeling overwhelmed. Tasks should be prioritized and broken down into manageable steps.
6. Seek Help: Discuss your emotions with friends, family, or a support group. Connecting with people can provide emotional support as well as stress relief.
7. Maintaining a balanced diet rich in whole foods is important since nutritional decisions can affect both physical and mental well-being.
8. Set Achievable Goals: Establish attainable goals and divide them down into smaller activities. Small triumphs along the way might help increase confidence and reduce stress.
9. Art & Creativity: Experiment with creative avenues such as art, writing, or music. Using your creativity to express yourself can be a therapeutic method to deal with stress.

MONITORING PROGRESS

1. Set clear and Realistic Goals: Define clear and attainable goals for your health or lifestyle changes. These objectives will function as checkpoints for your progress.
2. Maintain a Journal: Keep a journal to keep track of your daily activities, dietary choices, and any symptoms or improvements connected to your goals.

3. Utilize Apps and Technology: Use health and fitness apps to track your progress. These can monitor workout routines, dietary intake and even mental health.

4. Schedule regular self-assessment sessions to reflect on your path, celebrate accomplishments and identify areas for development.

5. measures and Measurements: Keep track of measurable indications like weight, body measurements or specific health measures that match with your goals.

6. Take regular images to visually document changes in your physical appearance, which will assist you in seeing transformations that may not be immediately evident.

7. Seek comments from friends, relatives, or healthcare experts. External opinions can provide important insights into your success.

8. Milestones: Recognise and celebrate tiny wins along the way. Recognising accomplishments increases motivation and encourages further effort.

9. Adaptability: Be willing to change your strategy based on what works best for you. Include some tactics in your regimen if they prove to be more effective.

FOOD AND SYMPTOM JOURNALING

1. Daily Meal Recording: Keep a record of every meal and snack including ingredients and portion sizes.
2. Include Beverages: Make a note of what you drink. Hydration can influence how your body reacts to certain foods.
3. Keep Track of Your Meal Times: Keep track of the times you eat your meals. This can aid in identifying trends associated with various times of day.
4. Keep a record of any physical or mental symptoms you have, such as changes in energy levels, mood or skin condition.
5. Find Triggers: Look for links between what you eat and the development or severity of symptoms. Identify probable triggers.
6. Consider the following Preparation Methods: Take note of how your meal is prepared. Grilling, steaming and frying can all affect nutritional content and digestibility.
7. Keep an eye on portion sizes because overeating can affect how your body processes and reacts to food.

8. Include Emotional Context: Keep track of your emotional state as you eat. Stress, happiness and worry can all have an effect on digestion and general health.
9. Record Supplement Intake: If you take supplements or vitamins, keep track of them. specific foods and supplements may interact with specific supplements.
10. Review your journal on a regular basis to detect patterns and trends. This knowledge can help you make dietary changes for better health and well-being.

TRACKING YOUR PSORIASIS JOURNEY

1. Document Flare-ups: Keep track of when and how long psoriasis flare-ups occur. Take note of the precise regions impacted as well as the severity of the symptoms.
2. Identify probable triggers such as stress, dietary changes or environmental factors that coincide with flare-ups.
3. Photographic Evidence: Take images of impacted regions on a regular basis to visually follow changes over time. This visual record can be quite useful for tracking development.
4. Medications and therapies: Keep track of the medications and therapies you use. Take note of your regimen's success, adverse effects and any changes you've made.
5. Lifestyle Factors: Keep track of your lifestyle choices such as nutrition, exercise and sleep patterns. These elements can have a major impact on psoriasis symptoms.
6. Weather Influence: Take note of how various weather conditions affect your skin. Some people may detect changes as a result of humidity, temperature or sunlight exposure.
7. Stress levels, emotional moods and key life events should all be recorded. Psoriasis is tightly linked to emotional health and analyzing these characteristics can show patterns.
8. Hydration and Diet: Keep track of your water consumption and nutritional choices. Staying hydrated and eating a well-balanced diet can help your skin's health.
9. Review your tracking data on a regular basis to find correlations and patterns. Make informed judgements regarding lifestyle changes and treatment approaches using this knowledge.